Embodied Spirit, Conscious Earth

Embodied Spirit, Conscious Earth

From Embryology to
Embodied Relational Spiritual Practice

Linda Hartley

tp

Triarchy Press

Published in this First Edition in 2024 by:
Triarchy Press
Axminster, England

info@triarchypress.net
www.triarchypress.net

Copyright © Linda Hartley 2024

The right of Linda Hartley to be identified as the author of this work has been asserted by them in accordance with the Copyright, Designs and Patents Act, 1988.

No part of this publication may be reproduced, stored in a retrieval system or transmitted in any form or by any means including photocopying, electronic, mechanical, recording or otherwise, without the prior written permission of the publisher.

All rights reserved.

A catalogue record for this book is available from the British Library.

Cover illustration: Brue Richardson

Print ISBN: 978-1-913743-99-4
ePub ISBN: 978-1-917251-00-6

Dedicated to the memory of my sister Susanne,

my mother Audrey Lily,

and my teachers Mary O'Donnell Fulkerson and Janet Adler.

Illustration and text permissions

Permission from Peter Hulton to reproduce images and text from Mary O'Donnell Fulkerson's *Theatre Papers – Language of the Axis,* is gratefully acknowledged. The papers were originally published by the Department of Theatre, Dartington College of Arts, Devon, UK. 1977

Permission from Raima Drąsutytė to reproduce her original drawings of embryology, anatomy and movement patterns, created to illustrate the text, is gratefully acknowledged.

Permission from Brue Richardson to reproduce her paintings 'Roots' and 'Spring' is gratefully acknowledged.

Body-Mind Centering® is a registered trademark, used with permission of the mark owner, Bonnie Bainbridge Cohen.

Contents

Preface 1

Part 1: What is Embodiment? 7

1: Conscious Embodiment 9
What Do We Mean by 'Embodiment'? 9
Conscious Embodiment of Movement 11
Three Moments 12
Embodiment and Dissociation 15
Returning Home to the Body 17

2: Coming Home to the Body 21
The Integration of Body and Mind 23
Visualisation – Somatisation – Embodiment 27
The Moving Self and the Inner Witness 29

3: Cultivating Embodied Presence 34
Stillness and Rest 34
Breath 35
The Language of the Body and the Language of Words 38
Presence – letting movement be just what it is 40
Transparency 42
Empty/Full 44

4: Somatic Movement, Somatic Imagination & Authentic Movement . 46
Attention and Intention 46
The Touch of Attention 49
Somatic Movement and the Potential to Heal 50
Working with Pain in the Body 51
Somatic Imagination and Dance-Making 53
The Discipline of Authentic Movement as Mystical Practice 56

  Healing 56
  Dance 56
  Mystical Practice 57
  Body as Sacred Vessel – Body as Prayer – Body as Offering 60

Part 2: Embodying Spirit 63

5: Embryological Beginnings 65
 Movement is Life 66
 The Dance of Conception – Feminine and Masculine 67
 Inside – Outside 72
 One Becomes Many, Many Are One – contents and container 73
 Coming into Relationship – self and other 76
 Bonding and Defence 80

6: Emerging into Form 82
 Bringing the Outside In 86
  Heart 87
  Nervous System 89
  Digestive Tube 92
 Organic Origami 94
 Unfolding to Verticality 95

7: Early Imprints 98
 Grof's Basic Peri-Natal Matrix (BPM) 100
 Womb Time, Eternal Time – BPM 1 102
 Paradise Lost – BPM 2 106
 Discovering Agency – BPM 3 108
 The Threshold between Life & Death, Joy & Anxiety – BPM 4 111
 Reflections 112

8: Meeting the World 116
 Emergence and Separation from the Ground of Being 118
 Relational Consciousness 122
 Mediating Inner & Outer through the Autonomic Nervous System .. 126
 Holding and Being Held 131

Part 3: Home and Ground 133

9: Body as Resource and Healing 135
The Grounding of Spirit in the Body.. 135
Trauma and the Upsurging of the Deep Psyche 139
Healing through Movement and Embodied Awareness.................... 141
The Discipline of Authentic Movement 142
Developmental Movement Therapy.. 144
    Cellular Breathing.. 144
    Navel Radiation 145
    Spinal Patterns 147
    Yield and Push 148
    Reach and Pull 149

10: Supporting Presence in Relationship.. 151
    Grounding.. 152
    Flexibility 152
    Centering... 153
    Boundaries 153
    Orienting in Space.. 154
    Negotiating Relationship 154
Balancing the Autonomic Nervous System 155
    Inside and Outside – the Cell.. 156
    Autonomic Rhythm 157
    Gestures of the Embryo 159
    Navel Radiation Pattern 159
Deeper In and Further Out 160
    Physiological Flexion and Extension... 160
    Birth... 162
The Support of Primitive Reflexes 163
Self and Other 164
To Summarise 168

Part 4: Communication and Connectivity 169

11: Cellular Body 171
- Whispering Between Cells 173
- The Emotional Brain and Psycho-neuro-immuno-endocrinology .. 177
- Energetic Pathways 179
- The Cell's Code of Three 182

12: Earth Body 184
- Whispering Between Trees 185
- We are Earth 187
- Earth as Witness 193
- Dancing with Earth Consciousness 198
- From Tribe to Individual to Interbeing 200
- Climate Change as Symptom 203

13: Collective Body 206
- Communication and Connection 209
- Embryonic Roots of Embodied Relational Spiritual Practice 213
- Global Expressions of Embodied Relational Spiritual Practice 215

Part 5: Endings and Beginnings 217

14: Transparency and the Aging Body 219
- Spirit Grows Younger as Body Ages 220
- Joyful Body, Painful Body 222
- Coming Full Circle – Witnessing the Return to Beginnings 226
- And Endings 227

Notes 233

References 239

Acknowledgments 245

Resources 247

Illustrations

Cover: *Spring*. Artist: Brue Richardson

Fig. 1.1: *Figure-of-Eight (a)*, from Mary O'Donnell Fulkerson's Theatre Papers
Fig. 1.2: *Figure-of-Eight (b)*, from Mary O'Donnell Fulkerson's Theatre Papers
Fig. 4.1: *Spheres in the Body*, from Mary O'Donnell Fulkerson's Theatre Papers
Fig. 5.1: *Dance of Conception*. Artist: Raima Drąsutytė
Fig. 5.2: *Cleavage – One becomes many*. Artist: Raima Drąsutytė
Fig. 5.3: *The Blastocyst*. Artist: Raima Drąsutytė
Fig. 5.4: *Hatching*. Artist: Raima Drąsutytė
Fig. 5.5: *Implantation*. Artist: Raima Drąsutytė
Fig. 6.1: *Three-layered disc with amniotic and yolk sacs*. Artist: Raima Drąsutytė
Fig. 6.2: *Three-layered membranous container and placenta*. Artist: Raima Drąsutytė
Fig. 6.3: *Heart and nervous system*. Artist: Raima Drąsutytė
Fig. 6.4: *Embryo becomes Foetus*. Artist: Raima Drąsutytė
Fig. 7.1: *Spirallic Diagram of the Basic Perinatal Matrix*. Linda Hartley
Fig. 8.1: *Two-layered cell membrane and cytoskeleton*. Artist: Raima Drąsutytė
Fig. 9.1-9.8: *Evolution of movement – Amoeba to Human*. Artist: Raima Drąsutytė
Fig. 10.1: *Physiological flexion and extension*. Artist: Raima Drąsutytė
Fig. 10.2 and 10.3: *Moro Reflex – two phases*. Artist: Raima Drąsutytė
Fig. 10.4: *Hand-to-Mouth Response*. Artist: Raima Drąsutytė
Fig. 10.5: *Asymmetric Tonic Neck Reflex*. Artist: Raima Drąsutytė
Fig. 11.1: *DNA and Heart Muscle as a Double Helix*. Artist: Raima Drąsutytė
Fig. 12.1: *Roots*. Artist: Brue Richardson
Fig. 12.2: *Barbara Erber, participant in IBMT Gathering, Dartington*. Photo: Linda Hartley
Fig. 12.3: *Spring*. Artist: Brue Richardson
Fig. 12.4: *Uprooted*. Photo: Linda Hartley

Preface

> *Our world today is in a crisis ... deeper and more widespread than any we have known throughout recorded history. Not only is the survival of the human race under threat, but we have created the potential for the devastation of our home, the earth, and all her inhabitants too. We perch precariously on the brink of catastrophic breakdown as the insubstantial structures of our society groan under the weight of ever-increasing pressures from within and without ... We pollute the earth, the air, the rivers and sea, the dome of sky that protects us from above, all in the name of progress, when all the time it is leading us into greater global danger.*
> (Hartley 2001: 33)

In January 1990 I began to write *Servants of the Sacred Dream* and wrote these words. They could have been written today, and each crisis that has arisen in recent years seems to be even worse than the one before it. The crises I was naming then have not only deepened but have also surfaced more fully into collective awareness. The crucial issue of climate change has finally become a mainstream concern, not only of climate scientists, environmental activists and lovers of the natural world, but of politicians and business leaders too, appearing in every newspaper, on every TV channel, and filling social media with articles and conversations. 'An idea whose time has come' – but now we are asking, 'Has it come too late?' Can we stop catastrophic climate change and species extinction, including our own?

The *polycrisis* we are now in the very midst of is collective and multi-dimensional; humanity has entered a collective initiation, a death-rebirth transition, which has long been predicted. Joanna Macy called it *The Great Turning* (Macy and Johnstone 2012). This is the time when the old way is dying, and we are now laying the blueprint for the new. This momentous transition has been going on for decades, maybe longer, and will take many more to fully complete, but it feels as if we have now entered the birth canal; we feel the pains of labour but are stuck, in the dark, no clear way through in sight. The feelings engendered at the early stage of labour can be of pain, fear, grief, betrayal, helplessness and hopelessness, feeling disempowered. We may feel like victims to greater forces working upon us.

What is needed for the birthing infant, and for humanity in the throes of birthing a new era, is a totally new way of being together and with the Earth. Can we accept the loss of the old ways, the pain of what is now, yield into the pressure and know that this is the way birth is? Acceptance of the pain can lead us through. Yielding might help us to discover the strength and power and will to do things better. We grieve for all we are leaving behind even as we must prepare for what is to come, being midwife to a death and a birth simultaneously.

Continued revealing of scientific evidence and *ongoing* activism will be required to force politicians and large corporate bodies to accept that change needs to come from the top down, to meet the creative and progressive changes from the bottom up that so many individuals, families, campaign groups and communities are already making.

It is thought by those in the intersecting fields of ecology and spirituality that several areas must be addressed in order to achieve the significant system change that is needed. The first and most fundamental is *spirituality and community*. Without this, without a deep sense of connection with each other and to that which is greater than all of us, changes in political, social, economic and agricultural systems will not hold.

I ask you, the reader, to hold this context in mind as we enter an exploration of the central themes of this book – *conscious embodiment* and *embodied relational spiritual practice*. I see these as forms of sacred activism that can also support and be part of the global movement towards a healthy society and planet. All intentions and actions which look towards a healthy and sustainable future can and must become the norm. We can seed intentions and actions that prioritise Nature over the unnatural; health and wellbeing over damaging practices; and creative community over destructive industry. And we must. This is our responsibility.

In this book I explore the process and practice of *conscious embodiment of movement*, which has been the core of my work over five decades of study, practice and teaching. But what does this have to do with the ecological and climate crisis we currently face? My experiences have shown me that when we are deeply connected to our own embodied being, we naturally come into deepened re-connection with the Earth-body out of which we have evolved and upon which we are totally dependent for life. When we listen to the language of our own body and learn from it what we feel and need, we develop the capacity to 'hear' the Earth speaking to us. Hearing Earth's messages, her teachings and her needs, we are inspired to give deserved respect and protection to the Earth and the natural world.

We are interdependent with Nature, not removed from it; we are totally reliant on water, air, sun, and the nutrients of the Earth herself. Without each of these elements, kept healthy, in balance and harmony, we can expect no life at all. In his seminal book *The Spell of the Sensuous*, David Abram (1997) helped awaken us to this reality. Writing about the deep interconnection we have with the natural world, he brought indigenous Earth-based wisdom into wider contemporary consciousness through a deep reflection on "the more-than-human world".

We are part of Nature. Our bones, the most resilient and lasting tissue of the body, are filled with the minerals of the Earth. Bones are the bedrock of the body, having the strength, beauty and constitution of marble if fluids and living tissue are removed (Juhan 1987: 92-3). Without our bony architecture we could not stand up and walk about on the Earth. Let alone build an aeroplane and fly across the world, or even sit at a desk to write.

Body fluids evolved from the ocean. We are part of the ocean and carry a part of it within us. From the moment of conception, we are bathed and held within an ocean of fluid that is a drop of the great ocean of the world; throughout life every cell of our body is surrounded by and filled with this fluid. It is the medium through which we breathe and are nourished, communicate amongst our different parts – cells and tissues – and maintain health and internal balance. The water of the ocean is our home, our protection and nourishment, and without it we cannot survive.

The oxygen we breathe is also essential to life. Trees and vegetation produce the oxygen that nourishes and energises us; they also absorb the carbon dioxide that we expel as waste and they are nourished by this. We live in exquisite reciprocity with the trees of planet Earth. This miracle of interdependence has genius within it. It is just one example of the complete interconnectedness that we and all species of the Earth partake in.

A television documentary showed a marvellous example of this, where dolphins and seabirds had developed a mutually beneficial system of attracting the fish that both feed on. Two entirely different species had learnt to work together to enhance the survival of both. And, of course, examples of reciprocal support are evident throughout Nature. James Lovelock revived the ancient Greek name *Gaia* for the intelligent, co-operative, interdependent, mutually self-sustaining systems of the planet and all its inhabitants (Lovelock 1991). When we become aware of the extraordinary complexity and subtlety of interconnectedness, it is hard not to see Gaia as an intelligent being with a consciousness of her own.

So, as we enter this exploration into conscious embodiment, I invite you to hold this wider context and questions about the consciousness of the Earth herself. Can we learn, from listening to the Earth as well as within our own body, what we each need to do to fulfil the responsibility we hold as custodians of this heartbreakingly beautiful planet that is our home?

Interweaving Arcs

The book will follow several interweaving arcs. Central to it are the embodied awareness practices of somatic movement, somatic dance and the Discipline of Authentic Movement; one arc follows development within this field of work from individual body-mind integration and healing to a conscious collective body that also embraces the potential for planetary healing. My own life and career path follow some of the strands of this field of work and some significant moments are touched upon.

Beginnings and endings of life mark another arc that unfolds from conception to dying. The evolving relationship between the matter of body and the mystery of Spirit through an individual's life is traced, as the theme of embodiment of Spirit is explored. We might also find ourselves asking 'where are we now in the arc of humanity's life in relation to our collective embodiment of Spirit, and of the consciousness of Earth herself?' In a spiritual emergency – a crisis of emergence into a new mode of consciousness perhaps?

Themes introduced in the early chapters will be returned to and explored more fully in later chapters, unfolding in overlapping waves just as with the development of the embryo, foetus and infant.

Nest

For more than a century and a half the wide and diverse field of somatic movement practice has provided a sheltered place where fledgling disciplines that invite conscious embodiment of movement, deep inner listening and the wisdom that arises from subjective experience, could develop, grow and flourish (Johnson 1995). This movement has often drawn upon ancient roots in global indigenous practices, integrated with modern scientific theory and research.

I think of the field of somatics as a *nest* within which nascent practices could be nurtured safely, within studios and circles of movers, partly hidden, protected from the premature gaze of unresponsive mainstream cultures. The field is largely peopled and led by women, along with a few significant male leaders, contributors and pioneers (Matthias Alexander, Moshe Feldenkrais and Rudolf Laban were notable early pioneers). Qualities often described as the 'feminine' have been able to find expression, enabling women and men who embody these qualities to become empowered in new forms of leadership, and enabling these qualities to become more known, strengthened and refined through research and practice. In this context the term feminine refers to relational and embodied modes of consciousness rather than to gender. These qualities include body and Earth consciousness; attuned relational awareness that engenders sensitivity and respect towards others and Nature; re-connection with the natural world and the indigenous perspective of mystical participation with the *web of life*. Of course, many men participate as deeply as women in this movement, and it is a union of healed masculine and empowered feminine values that we seek now.

In today's world we need to address simultaneously the climate and ecological crisis, and the re-balancing of feminine and masculine qualities within us and throughout the whole of human society; social and racial justice is part of this, as the dominant white and male culture of the preceding millennia has so often engendered inequality, injustice, oppression and harm to those seen as 'other' and to the Earth and Nature. It is time for the *somatics fledgling* to spread her wings and fly free from her nest, bringing the qualities that have been nurtured over many decades of research and practice more fully into view. They will be needed in both the healing of Earth and Nature from the climate and ecological crises, and the renewal of our human hearts, souls and bodies as we travel forwards. Somatic movement and Authentic Movement, practices that cultivate embodied consciousness, have many gifts to offer in this great work, some of which will be explored in these pages.

Linda Hartley
January 2024, Norfolk, UK

Part 1

What is Embodiment?

1: Conscious Embodiment

What Do We Mean by 'Embodiment'?

Spirit, consciousness, the life force moves through us from the very first moment of creation, the conception of a new being. Spirit becomes embodied, embedded in matter. The experience of embodiment is fundamental to being alive – matter enlivened by Spirit.

Speaking about Spirit is always a challenge. Each person's understanding, connection with and naming of that which we might call Spirit is utterly unique, intimate and often passionately held to. I will not try to define that which is by its nature ineffable, beyond definition, beyond words, beyond my own limited appreciation; but in order to orient to the matter of this book I suggest that the term Spirit could include what some might name Source, Universal Consciousness, Buddha Nature, God or Goddess – and all the names that different cultures and religions ascribe to this: Yahweh, Brahman, Allah, the Divine, the Sacred and more. I think what can be agreed upon is that each of these namings points towards an *invisible essence of life*, the Mystery at the heart of all religious and spiritual traditions. Qualities such as love, compassion, joy, awe, wisdom, beauty and bliss may be associated with it and a sense of deep connection, of union or non-duality, are present. The direct experience of Spirit, of the numinous, opens us to an awareness beyond our familiar and limited sense of self, to an experience beyond words that has the power to uplift, transform, heal and unite.

And what exactly do we mean by *embodiment*? Furthermore, what is *conscious embodiment*, for they are not quite the same? A young infant who does not yet have the capacity to self-reflect is embodied, but not in a way we might call *fully conscious*. The same for a stalking tiger or a dog excitedly chasing a ball. Embodied, most definitely yes – consciously so, well, not in quite the way we human animals think of it (though we will return to this question in later chapters).

A foetus, a new-born, a child and, perhaps for much of our lives, we adults are embodied but may not be fully conscious of this; we could speak of *pre*conscious (before consciousness arises), *sub*conscious (just below the threshold of conscious awareness but available to an invitation to rise above it) or *un*conscious embodiment (more deeply hidden from consciousness, often inaccessible to it, but nevertheless still present). We can engage with every aspect of life only because we are a body moved by Spirit, the life force flowing through us, sensing and feeling our way through myriad events and experiences that inform us constantly about our inner life and the world we inhabit. Spirit and matter inextricably linked. The depth of our conscious awareness of these flows of information varies from moment to moment and person to person.

Children who are nurtured into life with good enough support and care, held within a healthy balance of freedom-to-explore and safe boundaries, can retain the naturally embodied state that is every child's birth-right. A foetus, infant and young child swim in a world of sensory-motor interactions, feedback loops between movement and sensation which grow the young brain and enable the sense of a core self to develop (Stern 1985; Hartley 2004). To the extent that experiences of early neglect, abuse or trauma have *not* disrupted natural development, to this extent will a child be supported to grow into an adult with a sense of fully embodied presence.

Today *embodiment* has become a much talked about and valued process within movement disciplines, therapeutic practice of all kinds, spiritual approaches and culture more generally, but what is meant by this term? Traditional dictionary definitions may be useful as starting places, but limited in what they have to say on the subject: "to make (an idea etc.) actual or discernible"[1], or "to give a concrete form to; express, personify, or exemplify in concrete form. To provide with a body incarnate; make corporeal."[2]

When the term *embodiment* is used in psychotherapy, movement or spiritual practices, management training and the many other fields of learning and development which now draw attention to awareness of the body, often what is invited is the mind becoming aware of the body, the sensations, feelings and gestures it holds, and the patterns through which it expresses. Mind reflecting on matter – consciousness looking at the body. This is a deeply useful skill to learn, greatly enhancing any therapeutic or educational endeavour. Mindfulness Training (Kabat-Zinn 1990) and the practice of Focusing (Gendlin 1978, 1981, 2003) are two important practices that can help us to access the capacity of mind to witness, reflect on and influence bodily states and processes, leading us to a deepened connection with and perception of somatic and emotional experience. Yet there is more to it.

Conscious Embodiment of Movement

The field of *somatics* has a very specific approach that includes the cultivation of conscious awareness of bodily process, and also goes further. The *conscious embodiment of movement* is at the heart of this growing field of practice. Somatic movement practice cultivates the experience of consciously perceiving *from* and *through* the body as well as being conscious *of* the body and its states. Spirit is grounded within soma and they are wholly at-one, even if only for brief moments at a time. The original meaning of *yoga* – to yoke, or join – expresses the essence of this way of being.

Some believe that consciousness is created out of the movements of living forms: specific formative motions will create specific states of consciousness. Human embryonic development is expressed through unique gestures, which engender particular consciousness (Mott 1959; Blechschmidt 2004). Others believe that consciousness or Spirit pre-exists and infuses matter, so that matter becomes conscious through the act of conception (van der Wal online; Sogyal Rinpoche 1992). Or perhaps we can imagine that both processes weave together in the creation of each individual life.

After five decades of immersion in the practice of *consciously embodied movement*, I am drawn to review the question, 'what do we actually mean by embodiment?' The 'talking therapies' now use it widely, with the importance of the body in healing psychological wounds having been recognised. This has come about largely through insights from neuroscience and attachment theory (Schore 1994; Cozolino 2006), the development of somatic trauma therapies (Levine 1997, 2010; Ogden 2006) and the appreciation of mindfulness as a tool for growth, healing and the management of hard-to-treat conditions (Kabat-Zinn 1990). These three threads have woven together in recent decades to offer the bones and the lifeblood of a new paradigm for therapeutic theory and practice. This development has also been deeply influenced by, and sometimes grown out of, traditional and indigenous practices and worldviews that recognise and honour our intimate connection with Earth and the natural world.

In many approaches to psychotherapy and counselling the client might be asked to pay attention to what is happening in their body as they speak and explore difficult issues – what do they sense and feel there? The therapist might also have learnt the skills to track their own embodied responses and to use this information to help guide the work. This is foundational to body psychotherapy (Carroll 2009, Asheri 2009, Hartley 2004) and increasingly to other forms of psychotherapy. It is certainly a very welcome development, allowing a more truly holistic approach to therapeutic practice to emerge.

As a somatic movement practitioner and psychotherapist for many decades, as well as a long-time student of T'ai Chi Ch'uan and Buddhist meditation, my experience as therapist and teacher includes this approach of bringing attention to the perceived experience of the body. In addition to this, somatic awareness also embraces other perspectives, subtly nuanced and often hard to describe, as they exist largely before and beyond verbal language. This inevitably creates a challenge in finding language for the inner experience of being *consciously* embodied – fully present, in this body and this place, at this very moment in time. I offer a personal view, drawn from my own practice and teaching; I am sure readers will have their own ways of describing the subtleties of conscious embodied awareness practice, as inner experience is a deeply personal thing. However, I hope there might be a moment of recognition or clarification or disagreement that might provoke further reflection and even deepened practice for some.

I begin with three personal moments – three moments in my life when I was decisively stopped in my tracks, called to attend as awareness deepened, expanded, and a new mode of conscious embodiment arrived in me. (It is interesting to note the collective 'stopping' that was necessitated by the pandemic; the instructions to 'stay at home' and isolate from one another has indeed triggered new awareness – a closer connection with Nature for many and maybe, just maybe, a new embodied consciousness within our collective humanity is being born.)

Three Moments

> **One.** *I am about seven years old, walking home from school as I do every day, along Beach Road before turning into the crescent where I live. Suddenly and for no apparent reason I am stopped. My right foot stands firmly on the pale grey paving slab and the other hovers mid-step, just my toes touching the ground, keeping me balanced. I notice a crack that runs across the paving stone and the red-brick wall to my right. Beyond the wall is a narrow garden with a few small shrubs in front of the house, its white-framed bay-window in*

the centre. All of this enters my awareness in a flash. I seem to be suspended in this moment, weight falling through my right foot as the left reaches for the ground.

I am absolutely still. I recognise myself in this moment. I recognise that I am 'me' and I am standing on the grey concrete pavement by the low red-brick wall. The moment has a quality of clarity and simplicity. I am aware of myself – being here, being aware of my surroundings. The sun is shining, though not brightly – there is a layer of hazy cloud obscuring its brightness.

Here I am. A conscious inner self is born – a glimpse, a birth of my inner witness perhaps.

Two. *Now I am in my late twenties, a student from England living in the USA and studying Body-Mind Centering with Bonnie Bainbridge Cohen. Every day, with my fellow students, I embark on experiential journeys through my body's cells and tissues, discovering, expressing and clarifying movement patterns I had once known as a small infant then, in many cases, forgotten or overlaid with other patterns of movement. Sometimes totally new movement possibilities arise and these are embraced as an ever-expanding sense of myself evolves.*

We have a few days off and I am staying with a friend in Ithaca, upstate New York. I am to dance in an art installation he has created and while he is preparing the set I take a walk. I am walking along the edge of a road on the outskirts of the town, treading over the wide grass verge. The sky is blue and cloudless and the air is warm. An occasional car passes by.

Once again, I am stopped, made to stand still, made to feel my connection with the Earth, deep into the Earth. Both feet are placed firmly on the grass, lush green and long. I feel the soles of my feet soften and yield into the pull of Earth's gravity and I know myself rooted and connected to my Earth-home.

I feel completely and utterly whole, every part of me, every cell aligned and attuned in this moment. I am in my body, I am my body, fully present and alive. And I am deeply connected to the

Earth, I am the Earth. I feel the intrinsic inter-relationship between the tissues, fluids, minerals and breath of my body, and the elements of the Earth and space that hold me. I feel this as a living reality within me. I feel strong and powerful and rooted.

My conscious embodied self is fully present. My Earth-body is born.

Three. This time I am in my mid-thirties, in the midst of a transpersonal psychotherapy training in London. I have been travelling through the dark night of the soul, a time of deep pain and darkness in my life, of feeling lost and without hope. My soul is longing to feel connection with life again. I have driven out to walk in a beautiful and ancient wood that lies just west of the city. Relieved to be out of London for a while, I absorb the peace and the clean air of the woodlands. I am walking in a vast cathedral of beech trees that arc over me, their bright spring green leaves creating shifting patterns of light and shade, dappling the spring sunshine as it reaches the ground. The Earth beneath my feet is softened by layers of old leaves, mulched and dried out. Twigs crack underfoot.

As I walk beneath the corridor of tall and old trees, I can breathe more deeply, more freely. My body is settling into the rhythm of walking and the now familiar feeling of each step connecting deeply into the Earth. A joy begins to rise up in me, touching and opening my heart. I glance up into the green branches above me and once again I am halted mid-step, made to recognise the moment and all that it holds for me. The moment holds me, the trees, the sense of a presence that flows through both and fills me with a sense of my own deep feminine nature, the ground of my being. I am stopped. I am stilled, opened, looking upwards, with my feet firmly planted on the bare brown soil. I feel the subtle arc of my body, emerging out of the Earth and opening up towards the green light that filters through the trees.

In this moment I feel a new sense of expansion and connection – to the feminine ground within me and to a Divine presence that surrounds, embraces and runs through me. This presence, or energy, has the quality of the deep feminine, of Goddess, the

> *feminine aspect of Spirit. In this moment I am embraced by a conscious knowing of my Goddess-nature.*
>
> *My embodied connection to Spirit is born, or perhaps re-born, as I believe we all know this from our very earliest days but often lose connection as we grow, struggle to come into form and at times suffer deeply.*

These moments live in me today as clearly as when I first experienced them. What they each have in common is an expanded state of awareness; the senses become alive and perception acute; the sense of body in the environment is vivid, whole and connected to a world greater than my own inner experience. Whilst each moment heralded a new stage of conscious embodied awareness, they all had this in common as a foundation.

I learn from these experiences that moments of transition, of healing, new growth or profound learning are accompanied by states of deep conscious embodiment, as if such experiences can only land in us and be fully integrated if they are experienced by the whole of us, through all of our cells and senses.

Embodiment entails an active engagement with the sensations of being alive, being present, here and now, in this unique moment and place. As David Whyte writes: "Human genius lies in the geography of the body and its conversation with the world." (Whyte 2015: 78)

Embodiment and Dissociation

We cannot talk about conscious embodiment without naming the state of *dissociation* – a result of traumatic experiences that threaten our safety, our integrity and wellbeing, the people or things we hold dear and identify with, and our very life itself. Events that overwhelm our capacity to contain and process our emotional responses leave us without ground in our embodied sense of self. We struggle to orient in life and function in ways that are effective and creative; much suffering arises from living in a dissociated state. The vivid connection between bodily sensations, our sense of self and the wider environment, which is our natural state of being, is lost.

> *A specific moment imprints in my memory. I am walking along the water's edge with my brother. It's one o'clock in the afternoon, a summer's day by the sea. My denim jeans are rolled up and I splash barefoot through pools and gentle waves, feeling the sweet flow of*

cold clean water wash over my feet, feet that mould to the slopes and ribs of sand and small scattered pebbles as I step. There is sun and a gentle breeze, summer clouds flying high in the sky. All my senses are alert, filled with the sand between my toes, the easy swing of my seventeen-year-old legs, the comfortable feeling of my younger brother by my side, not speaking much but communicating companionship. Our silence is punctuated by the whirring of a helicopter above us, heading north, following the line of the shore.

I feel happy. The young man I love will be returning home soon and I am full of hope and optimism – my young heart nurtures a belief that all will be well.

Only later, much later, did I realise that the helicopter speeding up north hoped to rescue the same young man but could do no more than recover his body from the sea.

I could not have known all this as I walked along the beach that afternoon and heard the whirring helicopter blades cut through the air, and yet the sensory impressions of that moment were deeply imprinted in my consciousness. I was also not to know that this would be the last time for many years that I would experience the world with such vivid clarity. My life was divided in two – a life before, full of the intense immediacy of every moment, filled with bright colour and shape, sound, smell and touch, each moment a distinct and whole sensorily experienced world. And a life after, where I existed only partially, colours had faded, forms were barely noticed, sensations were vague or faint or distant to my touch.

Long before the words *embodiment* or *dissociation* entered my vocabulary, I knew what each was. The distinction between them was incised into my being in that instant when the helicopter flew over and I headed home with my brother for lunch.

Our wounds form us and often, if we are lucky and brave enough, they guide us to a path of both self-healing and work in the world. So it is no coincidence that I embarked early in my adult life on a path that would enable me to re-discover the experience of embodiment that I had been cut off from by this traumatic loss. My choice to leave academic studies when I was nineteen and instead study dance and movement practices was an intuitively felt, though as yet unconscious, choice to heal the split that had opened up inside me – the split between 'the life before and the life after'; between the feelings that tormented me within and the ghost of a self I had learnt to live through in the world; between a body that carried me well enough through life and a mind that was disordered and absent much of the time. The distance between these two – my authentic inner self and the remnants that I showed to others – was too painful to sustain forever. I had no choice but to find a path of healing if I was to survive at all.

I found dance, and through this a whole world of embodied movement practices opened up to me. As Peter Levine writes: "A gift of trauma recovery is the rediscovery of the living, sensing, knowing body." (Levine 2010: 356)

Returning Home to the Body

For fifty years, movement practices that support conscious embodiment have been at the core of my personal healing journey and a foundation for the work I do. During the 1970s Thomas Hanna re-introduced the Greek term *soma* into the vocabulary of a growing field of work that addresses consciously embodied movement practice. He described *soma* as "the body experienced from within" (Hanna 1970), subjective first-person perception, in distinction from the third-person objectified body that can be used as a commodity, misused, abused and related to as 'other'. Somatic awareness is a state of embodiment informed by sensations, feelings and movement impulses that we experience from within when we pay careful attention.

In *Touching Enlightenment,* Reginald A Ray writes:

> *To be disembodied is to be disconnected. The objectifying mind knows things only as lifeless concepts, as mental realities with no life, worth, or integrity of their own. When we objectify something, when we turn it into an object for our use, we lose touch with its reality as a subject...*
>
> *To be embodied, to be in the body, is to be in connection with everything ... To be in the body is to know our sense perceptions as opening out into a sacred world. (Ray 2014: 24)*

Reading this passage, it is clear the extent to which the objectification of the 'other', including the Earth and Nature, has led us down a path of dangerous disconnection and consequential damage.

Don Hanlon Johnson describes how the contemporary field of somatic practice was seeded by a few extraordinary nineteenth-century practitioners (Johnson 1995); their pioneering work has informed the rich evolution of many diverse and integrative approaches that we have access to today[3]. However, we can go back to philosophers such as Aristotle (Elisha 2011), as well as eastern Yoga and Martial Arts practices, to find earlier roots of the discipline that we now called *somatic movement*, the field of consciously embodied movement practice. The experience of embodiment is fundamental to being human and is a foundation to health, wellbeing and consciousness itself. We will explore this further as the book unfolds.

I would like to begin by describing the three movement disciplines that have formed the bedrock of my own learning and practice. Each offers a way to explore the invisible essence of Spirit through the tangible presence of the body. I feel extraordinarily blessed and privileged to have been able to study with three remarkable women, all pioneering teachers in the field of consciously embodied movement practices, though they might not always have been named in this way at the time. In the following chapters I would like to introduce some elements of their teaching that have informed my understanding and practice of this field of work, and hope I can honour the gratitude I feel for the opportunities they each gave me over my years of study and ongoing learning, practice and teaching.

After deciding to leave university and seek out a training in dance, I had the unexpected good fortune to find myself a student of Mary O'Donnell Fulkerson in the Dance Department of Dartington College of Arts, England. I had not heard of her work before and had no idea at all that I was about to step into a new era of dance practice in Europe, one critical thread of which had just appeared on this continent a year earlier with Mary's arrival as head of Dance at Dartington. I arrived as a student in 1974, totally naïve, uninformed, untrained, stepping into an unknown area of dance practice that proved to be, for me, the beginning of both a healing journey and a life-long career based in somatic movement practice.

Six years later, visiting the USA to study further, I embarked on a training in Body-Mind Centering with Bonnie Bainbridge Cohen. Study with Mary had prepared me well for the subtle and specific explorations of embodied anatomy and movement re-patterning that are a foundation of Body-Mind Centering training. In Bonnie's research and teaching I began to find fascinating answers to questions I had been asking, as well as new questions and a deepened and ever more subtly nuanced experience of embodiment.

And I was coming alive again in ways I had lost touch with for many years. The rift between my authentic inner self and my false self, riven through earlier trauma, could begin to heal.

Whilst studying in Amherst, Massachusetts with Bonnie and the Body-Mind Centering faculty, I was also introduced to the practice of Authentic Movement by students of Janet Adler. Janet was living and teaching in the town of Northampton where I also lived and, though I did not meet her at this time, Authentic Movement became a part of my personal practice. When, in 1993, I had the opportunity to study with Janet, I fell in love with her approach to teaching the Discipline of Authentic Movement. It seemed to offer a vessel that could contain all the practices I had been exploring – somatic, psychological, spiritual and creative.

From these three women I not only learnt about Release Work, Body-Mind Centering and the Discipline of Authentic Movement. I came to know myself more fully and deeply, to trust myself and my intuitive knowing, to honour my authentic experience as a guide in life, and to respect the *soma*, the embodied self, as a marvellous source of knowledge, wisdom, love, compassion, gratitude and prayer.

From Mary, as well as the somatic changes and creative inspirations I experienced, I learnt to let go of restrictive ways of learning. My experience of studying Release Work at Dartington was a process of *de-schooling* that enabled me to genuinely 'learn how to learn' – to research, develop, create and discover my own path in life and work (Hartley 2018: 358). As my body was being re-patterned into a more aligned and integrated expression of who I am, so too was my psyche being re-shaped into a whole new way of being and of experiencing myself.

Bonnie taught me to trust my own experience deeply, and from her teaching I learnt that there are multiple keys to awakening a person's connection to their inner self, to healing and to discovering an integrated wholeness of being. When we find the key that meets the need of *this* individual in *this* particular moment, healing happens and life flows with more freedom, vigour and purpose. Bonnie's teaching gave me an endless treasure of keys, which have continued to reveal themselves throughout my life.

Janet's teaching enabled me to further deepen trust in myself and my own intuitive knowing; to recognise and find language for the subtlest of experiences, thus enabling lost or hidden parts of myself to be integrated into conscious awareness; to see myself and another more clearly and communicate with fuller acceptance and compassion. Her teaching offered me an eternally evolving process of refining connection to self, to other, to Earth and to the Mystical, the Sacred.

Today, moving in the garden studio I recently had built at my home, there are moments when body memories awaken and I am once again in the studios of long ago, my younger self learning, embodying consciously for the first time. Studios with smooth wooden floors and sunlight streaming in. In particular, the Dance School at Dartington, where my journey began, comes back to me now. Moments of delight, of opening, spontaneously arise. Lightness. Freedom. Focus. Presence.

I am still there – young, a beginner, discovering the joy of mindful moving, of conscious embodiment – the grace, fluidity and even, nearly five decades later, the feeling of ease and freedom it brings. All of this still lives in me as embodied memory.

[A few months after this experience of re-living my time with Mary in the Dartington studio, she passed away. I had not known she had been ill at the time, but her Spirit had been so vividly present to me during that period of research in my studio. Now I understand that her consciousness was expanding, opening out and touching many of us who had known her, even as her physicality must have been contracting and turning inwards. Thank you Mary, for your precious life and teaching.]

2: Coming Home to the Body –

The dialogue between 'body and mind'

In this and the following two chapters I will be looking back at my own somatic movement journey, describing some key elements of embodied awareness practice as taught by my three primary teachers, Mary O'Donnell Fulkerson, Bonnie Bainbridge Cohen and Janet Adler. Among the many people I have studied with, these are the three whose teachings I have felt most drawn to and inspired to follow in depth, the three women whose work has had the most profound influence on my own developing practice. Over the years I have assimilated and integrated threads of their teaching and do not claim to give a thorough description of them here; I offer merely some glimpses into themes which run through each, connecting them as distinct disciplines within a shared field of practice, as well as defining differences. Anything that diverges from their original meaning or intention is due to my limited perspective or the ways that I have personally integrated the teachings I have received from them. Individually and together, they offer ways to explore the mysterious realm of embodied Spirit, an immanent spirituality, and also pathways into greater connection with oneself, with other human beings, the more-than-human world and the Earth body, Gaia, which is our home and ground.

As well as studies in dance, psychology, scientific enquiry and therapies emerging from western perspectives, each was also influenced by spiritual and healing disciplines with ancient, eastern and indigenous roots. These sources have informed, and been integrated into, their understanding and practice, and indeed into the proliferation of embodied practices that we are blessed with today. Mary's work was emerging in the cultural milieu of 1960s' America where teachers of Zen and other forms of eastern spiritual practice had arrived from Asia. Zen, in particular, had an influence on Mary and colleagues such as Steve Paxton. From her time living in Japan, Bonnie was deeply influenced by Zen, Aikido and the healing practice of *Katsugen Undo*, taught to her by Haruchika Noguchi. Janet's teacher, Mary Starks Whitehouse, was informed by Taoist philosophy in her development of Authentic Movement, and Janet herself researched deeply into the mystical traditions of both East and West (Adler 1999a). She has also spoken of an inner connection to a shamaness who has profoundly guided her work[1].

Mary had been a student and colleague of Marsha Palludan[2] in the USA, and had also been informed by the Releasing Technique of Joan Skinner. The importance of Mary's contribution to the emerging field of somatic dance and movement in Europe is sometimes overlooked or underplayed; here, in honour of her place as a pioneer, a leading light in the field, I let words from her early writings speak as openings into the exploration of conscious embodiment.

Peter Hulton, head of the Theatre Department at Dartington whilst I was a student there, and later principal of the College, created a series of Theatre Papers written by teachers and associates of Dartington from the 1970s onwards. I recently reviewed the papers written by Mary while preparing an article I had been invited to write (Hartley 2018) and could see how the seeds of all I had later come to study with Bonnie and Janet, as well as with my teachers of Buddhism and T'ai Chi Ch'uan, were present in Mary's teaching, sometimes in embryonic form and sometimes fully fledged. I could see how my path had been prepared during those many hours spent in the beautiful dance studio at Dartington, under Mary's inspired tuition. I will draw out some of the themes from her early writing, dating back to 1977 but just as relevant for us today, and then discuss how these threads, which were foundations of her teaching of Release Work, returned and were developed in my later studies with Bonnie and Janet.

These three practices feel very complementary to me; each can be explored alone or, if the practitioner wishes, integrated to deepen and enrich an exploration, as will be touched upon in some of the examples in these chapters. They can also be applied in somatic explorations of embryonic, foetal and child development, as we will see in Part 2. Sometimes a subtly different perspective or naming of a practice or an experience can open up new understanding and appreciation. In contemplating a particular theme through the lens of three distinct but related disciplines I hope this might be the case for the reader. More will be said about this in Chapter 4.

The Integration of Body and Mind

Thought and action together produce the whole self and neither can exist in isolation from the other. In order to use thought and action together a new language is employed. This is the language of the axis, not a language of words, but of experienced sensation.

(Fulkerson 1977: 2)

Release Work invites the use of mental imagery to inform bodily action. We begin with an image that is a simplified picture of the flow of movement through muscles, bones and joints; an image that encourages graceful ease, anatomical balance and efficient movement pathways. Information that is based on muscle action or anatomical alignment or whole-body movement patterning is "spoken silently throughout the body" (Fulkerson 1977: 3) to create real physical change over time.

The images trace intricate pathways within the body, threads of connection, cycles of energy that initiate easeful and graceful movement: circles, spheres and overlapping figures of eight; vertical lines of connection, integrating bones and joints, aligning the body with Heaven and Earth. The image is thought through the body repeatedly, often during an initial period of stillness, creating new sensations which begin to integrate into the somatic nervous system. In time, the image and the sensations it creates stimulate movement. As the movement unfolds it is informed by the anatomical information the image holds. Being in a relaxed and open state, the body is receptive to the new sensations that are generated, and through this receptivity new movement patterning can be experienced and integrated. A subtle resonance, a finely tuned balance, a sensitive alignment begins to develop through repeated practice.

In contrast to this, the memory of a distressing or traumatic event is also imprinted as image, sensation, feeling and movement impulses that might be blocked from full expression, or chaotic and disordered. Inviting or encouraging positive imagery that can stimulate new sensory-motor pathways can offer a more comfortable, safe and even joyful experience of the body and be a support towards healing and repair.

Now that we know of the presence of *mirror* or *empathy neurons*[3], we can understand more fully from the findings of neuroscience how this might work – how simply visualising a movement in the body, or witnessing another perform that movement, evokes activity in the very neurons which would be engaged were we to actively perform the same movement. Imagining movement with a particular set of directions, flows and qualities stimulates neural activity, which evokes related sensations and feelings. This creates new pathways within the nervous system through which movement can be initiated and sequenced, as well as profound shifts in the *quality* of the movement expressed.

Exploration of the Figure-of-Eight image from Release Work

An image from Release Work might begin in this way:

- ➢ Imagine a line, or flow of energy, down the whole of the back of the body, from the top of the thoracic spine to the back of the heels.
- ➢ Continue by circling underneath the feet and up the front of the body to the top of the sternum.
- ➢ Here, cross to the back of the body, up through the throat and neck; continue the direction of travel up along the back of the head, then down over the face.
- ➢ Below the chin, loop to the back again and repeat.
- ➢ The Figure-of-Eight image is visualised repeatedly until new sensations can be felt; these sensations become the impulse for movement to begin. The image can also be developed to include the arms, but we will stay with the simplicity of the single Figure-of-Eight for now.

In her teaching of Body-Mind Centering, Bonnie spoke of *imagination* as being more powerful than *will*. Imagination is used here, as in Mary's teaching, in the sense of the mind intending and guiding, through the creation of an image, a pathway or direction along which energy and movement are invited to flow. The imagination, or creative intention linked to specific anatomical structures in the body, opens up a potential for movement to flow in a new way – more freely or with clearer direction and integration, connecting parts, opening space, releasing holding. Imagination, as a function of intention, is a powerful tool to create such change.

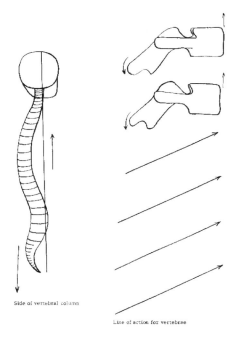

Figure 1.1: 'Figure-of-Eight – Action Flows Down the Back and up the Front', from Mary O'Donnell Fulkerson's Theatre Papers.

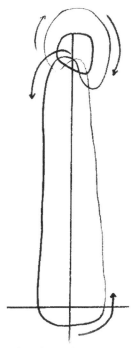

Figure 1.2: 'Up the Back and Down the Face combined with Down the Back and Up the Front', from Mary O'Donnell Fulkerson's Theatre Papers.

The Body-Mind Centering approach that Bonnie developed invites a deep and subtly nuanced experiential study of the body's anatomical systems, organs, tissues, fluids and cellular structures. The student learns to embody each in turn so that the experience of the body from within becomes an indwelling of a vastly complex and miraculous universe – precise, specific and detailed (Bainbridge Cohen 1993, 2008; Hartley 1995). That we can experience 'being' cell, or cell membrane, or mitochondria, or any of the organs, fluids or tissues of the body, may seem a strange idea to one who has not been introduced to this way of embodying, yet I believe we can all learn it with time and patient inner attentiveness.

This deep connection to our embodied being opens up the potential for very specific, focused therapeutic interventions or movement repatterning. Outcomes can often feel magical but they are clearly based in anatomical and physiological knowledge and skilful application. This information is "spoken silently throughout the body" (Fulkerson 1977: 3), often supported by the carefully chosen language and skilful touch of a practitioner, in a way similar to the process Mary describes; the anatomical detail engaged with in Body-Mind Centering practice is more explicit and detailed, but the act of thinking through the body is similar. Somatic teacher and author Sondra Fraleigh writes, "Consciousness is the embodied basis of mind. We function and live in a river of action, which is both physical and mental at once." (2015: 65)

Daniel Siegel has described all issues that bring clients to psychotherapy as being due to lack of *integration*, which is created by either too much *rigidity* and holding or too much *chaos*[4] (Siegel 2007: 198-9). In somatic work, too, we find exactly these same issues expressed through the client's movement patterns, body tissues and cells – a precise reflection of the condition of the psyche and vice versa. As creative change occurs in the body through consciously focused movement and bodywork, so too does the psyche adjust, releasing or integrating as needed. The somatic practitioner learns to recognise in which direction the client needs support and can adjust their interventions, whether it be through movement invitations or therapeutic touch or imaging through the body. Through the refining of imaginative intention, she attunes the quality of touch or movement intervention to encourage release where there is too much tension and rigidity, or connection where there is a lack of clarity and integration between and within the body tissues of the client.

Embodying the Figure-of-Eight image described above, sensations such as a release down the back of the body and a softening of the face, and a subtle activation up along the front of the body and a lengthening release up the back of the neck and head, might be felt. In time the new sensations invite movements to unfold spontaneously. Each person will move in their own unique way though their body is inspired by the same image, each improvising from the unfolding sensory-motor feedback loops that are being generated from visualising the image within the body.

The image encapsulates many anatomical details in a simplified form. The simplicity of the image gives the body lots of space to play and invent – *somatic imagination*[5] is cultivated. A freedom to invent new movement repertoire is invited, as well as a call to re-visit simple movements and gestures that we may not have practised since our infancy, such as rolling and crawling on the floor. Enormous pleasure and joy can be found within such freedom.

Working with the simplicity and holistic integrity of the image can be especially helpful for the dance maker seeking to source new material. However, when there is felt to be imbalance in the body – too much tension in one area, a lack of vitality, support or connection in another for example – the very specific work of Body-Mind Centering techniques can be helpful. *Muscle currenting*[6] can deepen the potential to re-pattern the muscle body towards more balanced use. Or focus on breath, tone and movement in the organs can help us discover the support and expressiveness their presence gives to movement and posture. Alternating these two approaches of somatic dance and somatic movement re-education can be helpful in integrating the body and also finding the freedom to spontaneously create new dance material.

Visualisation – Somatisation – Embodiment

The integration of body and mind is central to the practice of Body-Mind Centering, as the name implies. *Mind* in this context first includes thought, indeed both thought and imagination are used in the initial process of focusing attention on anatomical details, clarifying movement pathways and creating imagery within the body, as Mary also describes. *Mind* also holds a broader meaning that is closer to *awareness*; *embodied awareness* is central within all approaches to somatic work. Anchoring awareness in the body helps to still distracted thought, the restless 'monkey mind', and brings us into the present moment and place, to *presence*. *Embodied presence* is both an intention and a fruition of somatic practice and it develops as we learn to settle the cognitive mind – 'small mind' as it is sometimes referred to in Buddhist teaching – in the body. When this happens, mind expands into embodied awareness, which can be vast and global in its perception rather than specific and limited.

Bonnie has described three stages on the path towards full embodiment. First, *Visualisation* is the process, as described above, where we create mental imagery to encapsulate a complex store of anatomical and neurophysiological information; or hold the image of a physical structure – cell membrane, heart, psoas muscle, whatever it might be that we want to connect with – then "search to become aware of that part of your body." (Bainbridge Cohen 2008: 157)

This evolves into the second step, *Somatisation,* as we become aware of the sensations and feelings that are stimulated through the visualisation process. Rather than guiding, informing or intending as in the first stage, we are now witness to our inner experience; there is an inner witness, an awareness of the kinaesthetic, proprioceptive, interoceptive, touch and other sensory experiences that are evoked through attention focused in this specific way.

Bonnie describes the final stage of full *Embodiment* as "the cells' awareness of themselves ... a direct experience; there are no intermediary steps." (Bainbridge Cohen 2008: 157) Her description of fully embodied presence is sourced in cellular awareness and leads to "complete knowing ... peaceful comprehension". In her teaching she speaks of the need to first bring what is subconscious (mediated by the low-brain) into consciousness (mediated through the cortex); once a pattern has been made conscious, we can work with the processes of movement re-patterning. Then we let the new sensory-motor information drop back into the sub-conscious in order to fully integrate it into our way of moving and being.

Mary, too, writes of letting go of the image: "Finally, the image... becomes a forgotten source, a unity of body and thought. One no longer thinks the image but becomes it." (Fulkerson 1977: 14) From an imaginative thought process, mind broadens and deepens into embodied awareness. She describes this process in a way not unsimilar to Bonnie's three-fold description:

> *First I see it. I recognize the image. I begin to feel it with my other ideas and it remains strange, separate from me.*
>
> *Then I think it. I begin to let the image fall through the body. I apply the image to myself.*
>
> *Then I forget it. I have thought it enough so that the body knows. The image becomes a body state, a total situation. The image has fallen through the body.*
>
> *Then it happens. The body and the image become the same thing. There is no separation. Mind and body are in harmony. No longer is it an image. There is total participation.*
> (Fulkerson 1977: 94)

The Moving Self and the Inner Witness

Through Janet's evolution of the Discipline of Authentic Movement, the dichotomy of mind and body, and their integration, is further articulated. She speaks of an *inner witness* and a *moving self*, which we could see as particular expressions of mind and body. In Authentic Movement practice we might travel through many inner landscapes of experience, many relationships between the inner witness and the moving self; the Discipline offers a way to explore this relationship and bring them gradually towards a place of greater integration. It is fundamentally a discipline which supports the cultivation of an ever deepening and evolving inner witness, held within the safe container of relationship with another person, the outer witness.

The mover closes his eyes as he enters the movement space; this allows attention to focus more fully on his inner world with less distraction from visual and social cues coming from outside. It also allows the often-dominant visual sense to quieten, allowing the other senses to awaken more fully; this can enrich the experience of the inner life immeasurably. The outer witness is the one who sits at the edge of the space with eyes open, paying attention to the mover and also to all that she is experiencing in the mover's presence. She takes care of the safety of the mover and the time boundaries for the session. Through the attentive, non-judgemental and compassionate presence of the outer witness, the mover's inner witness can gradually develop. More will be said about the relationship between inner and outer witness as we go on.

The cultivation of the inner witness is closely related to the body-mind integration quest, articulated within a framework that focuses on deepening connection: with self, with other, with the natural world and with the Mystical – that which is beyond our ordinary comprehension, cannot be fully known and named through the cognitive mind. We might start from a place of disconnection and an 'absent' inner witness but gradually, through attending with care and being seen clearly by the outer witness, the inner witness emerges and strengthens. There are various steps in the evolution of the relationship between the inner witness and the moving self that I have experienced and witnessed in my own personal and teaching practice; they can be viewed as a process or continuum of happenings. As a mover's inner witness gradually develops, over time, the following might be experienced (and there may be more).

- The inner witness is absent, asleep, unconscious.
- Thoughts might distract us and halt the movement.
- Or the body might take over and movement happens outside of conscious awareness. A subtle dance is always at play in the body, but below our conscious awareness for much of the time. It might emerge into expression when the inner witness is absent, revealing a new path of movement. In this case, a great amount of sensory information is still being registered subconsciously by the cells, nervous system and brain. Awareness of this can be brought to consciousness later, during the time of recalling and sharing experiences with the outer witness. The outer witness's recalling of the movement supports the awakening and development of the mover's inner witness.
- The mind might have been distracted for a while, as the body continues its path of movement unnoticed. As mind returns to the body we can be grateful for this moment as the inner witness revives; noticing what the body is doing, we might slow down and discern what is essential in this moment, what is the impulse that is guiding the movement, and allow this to unfold with deepened attention: *the head turning side to side, fingertips tapping on the floor, or the sensation of weight and pressure along the front of feet and knees and forelegs as I kneel; the experience of stillness as I slow down and arrive in my centre.*
- A part of the personality such as the inner judge, critic or analytic mind takes the place of the inner witness. This can feel paralysing to the mover if the dynamic has not been made conscious and sufficiently de-toxified. As we learn to recognise and witness the presence of the judge or inner critic, we come closer to experiencing the inner witness as a place of clear, accepting, non-judgemental, compassionate awareness. It emerges as an expression of the core self rather than of a part of the personality such as the critic.
- The mind/intention leads and directs the body. This relates to what Mary Starks Whitehouse described as the experience of "I move" (Starks Whitehouse 1979: 82), an intentional impulse that could be what she referred to as a 'functional' movement; for example, a mover might want to stretch his body to feel more at ease or shift his

position to relieve pain. A primary focus on the physicality of the body, carried out with conscious awareness, is part of the practice and might, when we attend with concentration and care, lead to an opening into other layers of experience. Everything is welcome; the focus is on paying attention so that we can feel what is essential within the moment and notice when other layers of our being begin to reveal themselves.

- The imagination initiates movement and the inner witness follows, personal images or stories generating spontaneous movement journeys that are witnessed as they unfold.

- A subtle feeling or strong emotion might initiate movement. If the inner witness is present the emotions can be expressed safely and also contained; recollection after the moving time enables completion and integration of the experience into consciousness and within relationship to the outer witness. If strong emotions overwhelm the inner witness, it might not be safe to continue moving spontaneously, with eyes closed; it will also be more difficult to integrate the experience into consciousness afterwards. The careful attention of the outer witness is important in keeping the practice safe for the mover.

- The body may lead, initiated by kinaesthetic, sensory or energetic impulses that are not censored or inhibited by the mind; the inner witness follows, tracking where the body goes and what is sensed and felt. The inner witness pays attention to the movement as it happens, registering the gestures, sensations, sounds, feelings and other experiences that emerge. Movement can be felt to arise spontaneously from the personal or collective unconscious, or it may be an expression of the Mystery beyond our known world. The experience of "I am moved" becomes known (Starks Whitehouse 1979: 82).

- Sometimes the inner witness is clearly present in the body, at a particular location, and the energy of this focused attention initiates movement there, evoking sensation and feeling. The T'ai Chi masters of old said that where the mind-intent goes, there Chi (energy) follows; where Chi flows, there movement happens (Liang 1977: 70). Movement arises when conscious attention is focused, or arrives, at a particular place in the body; energy is activated, or allowed to flow, and the movement of energy can be experienced directly and consciously. Perception of sensation becomes ever subtler, until the flow or tingling or vibration of energy is central in awareness.

> At times, by grace, the inner witness and the moving self are completely at-one. Intimate connection between the inner witness and the moving self allows us to be fully conscious within the experience of embodied presence, without thoughts that separate mind and body and distract from the moment. Full embodiment, *unitive presence* is experienced – we are fully present, in this very place at this moment in time – there is no separation between the moving self and the inner witness. We arrive in a state of *at-oneness* within ourself that can open us to an experience of connection and at-oneness with that which is greater than our personal self – a state of embodied presence that is both full and empty, and invites an opening to the Numinous, the Mystical, the Sacred.

All of these experiences are possible; none are 'wrong'. We can see them as points on a continuum of learning, part of a process of cultivating our inner witness. Always the intention is to become as conscious as we can to the fullness of our experience in the moment, whatever it may be, without judgement. A clear, accepting and compassionate inner witness develops in this way. If we begin or arrive in a place of 'absent' inner witness, when consciousness returns we are simply grateful for this return to presence, and carry on. These ways of being in relationship with oneself can also be mirrored in the relationship between the mover and their outer witness.

Embodied experience is, by virtue of its non-verbal nature, almost impossible to fully capture in words; our personal naming of experience may vary, depending on the paths we have taken in developing our practice. Hearing the words of Mary, Bonnie and Janet, I feel that they are touching upon similar areas of experience, languaged differently and coloured by the paths that have led them there. In my personal practice it seems that full embodiment can take on many flavours but there is an essential nature which runs through all: movement and image, body and mind, moving self and inner witness become completely at-one in an experience of full, conscious embodiment, free of distracting thought, present in the moment and open to invitations from the mystical as well as the earthly and human realms.

I hope the reader will take all I write here not as some attempt at a final truth. If you are already a practitioner of some embodied awareness practice, perhaps the ideas offered here will invite you to reflect, research and maybe explore with others to further your own practice and understanding. And if you are not yet familiar with such practices I hope that something in these pages will trigger your curiosity to experience them for yourself, perhaps with an experienced practitioner to guide you.

3: Cultivating Embodied Presence

Stillness and Rest

> *Resting ... find the possibility of listening to the body. Experience the inner complexity. Breath is easy. Weight is allowed to fall – given to the floor surface. Develop the quality of patience. In stillness, waiting is not necessary. Stillness is a positive state, complete and full in its expression. Do not wait for the end of stillness. Stillness is not an absence or expectation of movement. It is stillness.* (Fulkerson 1977: 51)

I love these words, their wise advice. In our busy modern way of life it can be hard to give ourselves permission to be deeply still and find truly nourishing rest, without the expectation of something else to come. The process of finding stillness, first of the body then increasingly of the mind, is fundamental to somatic practice and central to the experience of embodied presence.

To work with an image in Release Work we often begin in the 'constructive rest position', lying on the back, knees bent and soles of the feet on the floor, arms resting where they are most comfortable – alongside the body or with hands resting on belly or ribcage. Many somatic practices begin in this way. Although other positions, and sometimes simple repetitive movement sequences, can also be a starting place, this position allows the bones to align, breath to flow more easily and weight to be fully supported by the ground. From here we *listen* deeply to the body – which simply means we open our awareness to the stream of sensory information that is constantly reaching our central nervous system from all parts of the body and through all sensory channels. As we listen, more and more of this endless symphony of sensory messages becomes audible – and we come to know our selves more intimately as our felt-sense awakens.

Settling deeper into physical ease and rest, the nervous system becomes receptive to the invitations that the image suggests. In Body-Mind Centering practice this might include receptivity to the touch of the practitioner's hands as well as their words and the images they invite. It might include experiencing the support of the Earth through resting in different positions: for example, lying on the belly then the back to re-experience the total body support of the *tonic labyrinthine reflex,* which draws the new-born to bond completely with the Earth-mother's body (Bainbridge Cohen 1993:127). Or it might be that an alternation of rest and easeful movement allows a deeper and deeper letting go, as positions are found that encourage fuller yielding of weight into the ground.

In Authentic Movement, too, a mover begins by listening inwardly, often in stillness. Paying attention without expectation or intention for anything particular to happen, we begin to notice impulses playing below the surface of everyday consciousness. In this Discipline we enter with an awareness that is open to whatever might arise, be it movement, stillness, gesture, sometimes sound. Out of the stillness impulses to move might arise as sensation, feeling, image or the subtle perception of energy. They might come from the personal conscious – I, myself, intending a specific movement; or from a personal, transpersonal or collective source that is not yet conscious – messages from beyond our everyday consciousness that are calling for our attention. We follow these impulses, "like following a pathway that opens up before you as you step." (Starks Whitehouse 1963: 53) We witness whatever unfolds.

When we can inhabit stillness, not waiting for something else to happen but being fully present within it, we can come to know its textures more completely – bodily sensations, the quality of energy, traces of a feeling, a memory awakened by inner taste or smell, or experiences of bliss, love, awe, joy and emptiness – all of these and more can become known as we inhabit stillness fully. And out of it, movement might arise without effort or intention, often surprising us with its unexpectedness.

Breath

> *The image is (then) made the centre of attention. The image is recalled on every breath-out whilst the image falls out of conscious thought on the breath-in. First one thinks the image and then the image rests. The body remains still until action is demanded from the image itself.* (Fulkerson 1977: 14)

There is no forcing of the image or of the movement. There is space for rest within the initial engagement with the image. We focus, create, visualise the image, then the image rests. We rest, we let go. An invitation with every breath to simply be, to be present without thought or activity. What a gift this is for us amidst our busy lives! This alternation of focusing during the out-breath and resting on the in-breath is also used in some meditation practices. There is deep wisdom in these simple instructions.

An alternation of active attention and rest lays down a foundation for the rhythm which is crucial to our wellbeing at all levels. The *autonomic nervous system* regulates these rhythms within our body and psyche, alternating rest and activity throughout hourly, daily, monthly and yearly cycles. Thus, the practice of breathing as described by Mary (and others) might support the re-balancing of the autonomic nervous system. As well as opening the psyche and soma for creative inspiration, the practice can aid in releasing stress and healing the psyche-soma in the resolution of trauma and post-traumatic stress disorder. When in a restful *parasympathetic* state, deep healing and change can occur[1]. (We will return to this in later chapters.)

Attention to the breath is used in many practices, both healing, therapeutic and spiritual, to help still the mind and body. The breath is also a bridge between what we are conscious of at any moment in time and all that is not yet known. Traditional psychological theory used the term 'the unconscious', but in contemporary thought the use of a noun that suggests some 'thing' that exists somewhere within us is considered to be too static a concept. Consciousness is a process not a state or a 'thing'. That which is not yet known, which is unavailable to our consciousness in a particular moment, can sometimes become known when careful attention is paid – to our movement expressions, our dreams, our feelings, in deep reflection or meditation for example. From a traditional psychoanalytic perspective, that which is not yet conscious consists principally of suppressed, repressed, forgotten or not yet experienced aspects of our psyche; material that belongs to the shadowy world of personal, cultural and collective history lives there, often profoundly influencing our thoughts, feelings and behaviour. In the Discipline of Authentic Movement, as in transpersonal psychology, 'all that is not yet known' also includes our unrealised potentials, the unknown possibilities of life, experiences of the Sacred, of Spirit, and so much more of the world and life that has not yet entered our conscious awareness. But perhaps it might do so when we attend with care and love, and when we breathe with mindful attention to the sensations that breath generates.

Our breathing mechanism consists of organs and muscles that are co-ordinated by the autonomic nervous system, beyond conscious control; it also engages groups of muscles which can be controlled consciously through the somatic nervous system – we all know how to hold our breath for a limited period of time, or breathe more deeply, slowly or quickly at will. Breathing functions at an autonomic level throughout our lives, fortunately, so that we carry on breathing when our attention is focused elsewhere; we can also control it to some extent through conscious intention. And our emotions, thoughts, environment and stress levels all influence the quality, depth and pace of our breathing; this happens beneath conscious awareness unless we bring mindful attention to it.

Because of this unique place as bridge between what is conscious and all that is not yet known, awareness of breath can open access to material that has been hidden – the feelings, memories, dreams and images that are normally below the threshold of conscious awareness, as well as the potentials that have not yet been touched and explored. For the dance-maker, an endless store of new material becomes available. As Mary writes:

> *This has the effect of bringing forth an ability to penetrate the barrier between conscious and unconscious thought. A day dream has the full presence of a night dream. Deep feeling can pour outward, even surprising the body with unusual perceptions. One discovers continually that things are not as they seem.*
> (Fulkerson 1977: 32)

Mindfulness of breath can support relaxation and nurture a para-sympathetic way of being; this cultivates the receptivity needed for the image, thought or creative idea to meet with hidden, deep-rooted and unconscious patterns that are not helpful to us. These might be inefficient movement and postural habits, destructive behavioural patterns or negative emotional and thought processes; as all of these are intimately connected in what Wilhelm Reich called a 'functional unity' (Reich 1970: 241-2), change at one level can affect all others. The somatic movement practitioner works primarily through the body to reach the mind, emotions and behaviour.

The Language of the Body and the Language of Words

> *The language of the body can be found below the language of words. Deep feeling, clear perception, the center of an idea, all these happen underneath words on a sensory level of experience. The world we call real is only a fragment of the whole world. Tremendous participation is possible between a body and a thought. The happenings underneath words can speak directly to anyone who patiently listens.* (Fulkerson 1977: 32)

When a dancer performs from the fully embodied place that Mary, Bonnie and Janet teach and write about, so much of this hidden sensory world can be intuitively perceived by the audience. Much is spoken without words and the person viewing can participate actively as their own feelings, perceptions, ideas and images are evoked. In my early years as a dance-maker and performer I was often surprised by the comments of audience members who perceived so much of the material that had arisen during, and had informed, the process of creating but was not present in the performance in any explicitly visible way. The movement still carried the layered processes that had gone into its creation; the language of the body held the memory and the information, without the need for words or explicit gestures. This is fundamental to artistic practices that speak through the non-verbal media of movement, image and sound to convey so much that cannot be easily put into words.

The Discipline of Authentic Movement offers a sacred space for healing and mystical practice as well as creative exploration, and articulation of the relationship between the language of the body and the language of words is a central concern. In this discipline we pay ongoing attention to finding words that will not only describe closely the embodied experience but might also enhance and deepen connection to the movement experience, to the mover's inner self and to their relationship with an outer witness. The mystery of the ineffable nature of embodied experience is fully acknowledged and embraced, even whilst we seek to find language that is clear of projection, interpretation and judgement, words that speak directly to our experience in the moment so that we may recognise its many layers – movement and stillness, sensation, feelings, images, memories, thought. In this, we may come to see our self more clearly.

The language of words more than anything else has enabled the modern world to develop. Without it we would not have electricity, cars, computers, aeroplanes or any of the multitude of things that make our lives easier in so many ways, more interesting, faster – but also more damaging to the health of the planet and humanity as a whole in so many other ways. It is the greatest 'mixed blessing' we have been able to create.

As psychologist Daniel Stern describes, the development of language enables the young child to share their internal universe with others – *I feel sad, I am angry, I love you* – so making it possible to be both separate and together in new and intimate ways. But it also drives a wedge between the pre-verbal, global world of experience that is our sensory-emotional-imaginative inner self and the world as represented by language. All that cannot be expressed in words and shared with another is relegated to the unconscious shadow – what Stern calls the 'disavowed self' develops, hidden, unknown and unexpressed (Stern 1985: 227-9). We may grow into adulthood knowing and expressing only a fraction of who we truly are.

And it is not only from other human beings that the development of language distances us. We become separated from Earth and Nature, from the 'more-than-human world'. We lose our innate connection as embodied creatures – made from the same elements of earth, water, air and fire – to our ground and home. David Abram articulates so eloquently the evolution of language from expressive sound, to spoken stories that are embedded in Nature and a sense of place, to hieroglyphic (pictorial) representations of things, to the abstract symbols that we know as letters and the written word today. This evolution has uprooted us from a deeply felt connection with the natural world (Abram 1997, 2017).

Finding a way to re-language our experience so that we can begin to heal this rift is close to the heart of the Discipline of Authentic Movement. We take time to find the words that will connect most intimately with our inner experience of our movement or our witnessing of another's movement. When the right word is found there is an 'aha' moment, a recognition, a sense of integration; a process that has felt incomplete can be resolved. When these words are shared with others and land fully, there is a deepening of connection between the participants as the truth, the authenticity of the experience and the language, is mutually recognised.

It is a rigorous path that takes many years of careful practice, unpicking the places where we habitually project onto another from the obscuration of our own personality and history; or tend to judge or interpret our own or another's movement through lack of conscious attention and conscious speaking. As we take the time to do this there are many rewards: hidden layers of experience can be unfolded, enriching our sense of self and our connection to others; that which is invisible within us becomes more discernible as the density of the personality clears and transparency emerges. As we practise the ritual of moving and witnessing, followed by the ritual of speaking and listening with others, the lived experience of a conscious embodied collective can grow; awareness of our participation in the *web of life* is cultivated as we open our heart and our senses to all that is beyond our personal and limited experience of self. When awareness of this participation becomes a living reality within us, we come to appreciate how attending to the healing of our own wounds contributes, in some small but nonetheless meaningful way, to the healing of the whole – the collective body and the planetary body.

Presence – letting movement be just what it is

> *Action means only what it is. Participate in action without attaching interpretive evaluations. Become very comfortable with physicality. The body speaks of the body.*
>
> *… Working comfortably allows separation from the question of "What does it mean?" to "What is now?"* (Fulkerson 1977: 84)

When, in the mid-1970s, Mary's non-interpretative approach to dance-making arrived in the UK it was new, radical for the time. Modern dance based on Martha Graham's inspiration was in vogue, with *The Place* in North London having recently opened to train young dancers in her technique and a symbolic, narrative approach to choreography. Mary's work attends to the cultivation of full presence within the physical gesture; the body, its movement or gesture, contains the image or story because of the full immersion in its reality that has gone before. Movement emerges spontaneously from this immersion:

> [D]ancers find a body state in which they become the images of the story. The gesture does not pretend to be the story. Accepting being the story comes before any gesture. Deep participation in the image yields the process. Deep participation yields the inside of the image from which the body state is formed. (Fulkerson 1977: 89)

I have a clearly embodied memory of being invited by Mary to create a 'Horizon Dance'. We were led out to a small hill behind her cottage at the edge of the Dartington College grounds. It looked out upon a wide view of the surrounding countryside. The instruction was simple. Be witness to the horizon all around; allow the perception of the horizon to come into the body, to be absorbed until it *becomes* the body and the body becomes the horizon; allow the body to move with, then from, then *as* the internalised image of the horizon. We opened senses to the panorama of the distant Devon hills, our feet received the touch of grass on hard earth, our skin the soft breeze and a hint of early summer warmth. Letting our cells internalise all we saw and felt, we allowed the horizon within to move us.

Back in the studio we were invited to re-create the Horizon Dance. I remember this so vividly. My body was choosing how and where to move – along the length of the dance studio wall in one long sequence of arcing movements. They are still imprinted in my cellular memory, the arcs, sweeps and turns, stretches and spirals. There was such deep pleasure in *being* the horizon and this embodied memory lives in me still.

Mary writes of this practice:

> *When I go to the ocean and see the line where the water meets the sky. I walk on that line, over it, across it, floating, stepping carefully, sometimes in water, sometimes in air. With my new body I can step into air or water without being dropped or drowned. I open my arms and become that line. Half of me is water, half air ...*
>
> (Fulkerson 1977: 89)

In her evolution of the Discipline of Authentic Movement Janet has arrived at a similar place of relationship to image and story. In the early years of practice, a mover might spend much time unfolding material related to her personal history – lost or hidden memories, images, stories, as well as archetypal and mythic journeys might arise out of unconsciousness and be expressed through movement, seeking to be integrated into an expanded consciousness. In this way the sense of self deepens and the mover recovers parts of herself not previously known and expressed, perhaps repressed at some earlier time in her life. This is the psychological and healing work that forms a foundation of the practice, where image and story, archetype and myth might help the mover to find meaning in her movement journeys.

At some point, usually after many years of practice, the mover might come to a place where enough of "the density of her personal history"[2] has been cleared, so that she no longer feels the need to keep returning to the realm of image and story to find meaning in her movement. The personal narrative does not need to be indefinitely repeated and elaborated. Interpretation is not needed. The practice of presence becomes primary.

When we arrive at this place in our evolving practice it is enough, and essential, to pay the fullest possible attention to the arising of each moment – witnessing the precise and detailed unfolding of the movement, the sensations, feelings and energetic phenomena that accompany it. The movement itself reveals the complex layering of experience which has given rise to it and which it is an expression of, but not a symbol for. The movement is what it is, pure and simple. Insight may arise spontaneously but interpretation or analysis are not needed.

The mover, together with their witness, unfolds the moment to discover the many layers of experience, searching for the words that resonate most closely and intimately with all they know about the moment. Taking time to do this through verbal exchange after the moving time, the mover might discover that the movement itself is an opening, a portal, an invitation into an experience of that which is greater than her personal self. At times the witness might participate in a shared experience of expanded consciousness, as a *unitive state* arises in both (Adler 2002: 209). In this way, the discipline of attending to the intimate details of a moment of movement can open both mover and witness to a state of shared mystical experience.

Transparency

> *Transparency is a quality which is present when people are moving with full mind and body concentration upon the physicality of any moment ... Direct contact of mind and body are revealed. Energy is seen naked. It is not the personality alone which becomes visible. It is the total mind and body self. When mind and body are united the result is a very simple, direct expression of intention. One can see through the whole person to find this intention. The person becomes transparent.* (Fulkerson 1977: 93)

In dance performance, the intention within the movement can become known by the audience without the intermediary processes of symbol and interpretation. The audience are invited into a state of presence, of mind and body integration, as they witness the nakedness of the movement. Watching dance can be transformative for the audience, as it is for the dancer. Of course, there are many skilled and beautiful dancers who can convey this experience whilst also describing symbolic narratives through their dance; if they have the power to transform the audience, they are most likely dancing from a place of full embodiment that reveals the transparency of the gesture. In Mary's work the intermediaries of symbol and interpretation are pared away to leave us with the naked truth of the body moving.

Transparency is a quality which arises with deep attention to the moment in Authentic Movement practice. At times the witness sees the mover clearly and through this, the mover is enabled to see himself more clearly. Both are fully engaged in the moment – present, aware and attentive to the fullness of their own experience. Intuitive knowing becomes possible. The invisible is made visible. Janet describes how it is through seeing the other clearly that the witness also comes to see herself:

> [S]elf-witnessing is transformed after truly seeing another as she is. It is as though there is now a reversal. In the same way that being seen by another originally enabled me to see myself as I am, in a further sweep of the spiral, seeing another as she is – loving her – enables me to see myself as I am. (Adler 1999: 154)

The idea of making the invisible visible through the practice of moving authentically was present in Mary Starks Whitehouse's original work: "[M]ovement is a way to get in touch with yourself – the invisible part." (Starks Whitehouse 1963: 31) In developing the practice of what came to be called Authentic Movement, Starks Whitehouse was deeply influenced by Jungian psychology; what she named "the invisible part" consisted largely of all the unconscious and unexpressed content of the psyche, which could be made visible through embodiment in expressive movement. She was also informed by Taoist philosophy and we might assume that embodiment of the Mystical was part of what she intended here, though maybe it was not so explicitly central to her approach as the psychological. Janet developed this aspect more fully in her evolution of the Discipline of Authentic Movement, the 'invisible' coming to signify all that is not yet known in our experience, both within and around us; this can include the Numinous, the Sacred, the Mystical. As Bonnie Morrissey and Paula Sager write, "Mystical experience is a realm of subjective communion with that which is invisible, the infinite unknown." (Adler, Morrissey and Sager 2022: 36)

The many layers of complexity that are a human being, the total expression of the psyche – including body, feeling, thought and imagination – and Spirit may become visible in moments of deep, full and clear attention to the moment.

Bonnie describes the process of transparency in this way:

> *I see the body as being like sand. It's difficult to study the wind, but if you watch the way sand patterns form and disappear and re-emerge, then you can follow the pattern of the wind or, in this case, the mind. I knew long ago that what I was seeing on the physical level was only ten percent of the whole picture of what I was seeing. Mostly what I observe is the process of mind.*
> (Bainbridge Cohen 2008: 11)

Soma is the embodied expression of psyche. Psyche is the invisible flow of energy and information that underlies soma. Through attending, with love, to the intimate intricacies of embodiment, the whole person can become known and Spirit may be revealed.

Empty/Full

> *One waits as if empty through the whole process of this work and it is such availability that allows for the recognition of possibility. The sense of absence is not passive. It has to do with the recognition of multiple possibilities ... This empty state is very active. Being absent in this way is being fully present.* (Fulkerson 1977: 95)

When a mover arrives in a place of fully embodied presence, of transparency, an altered state of consciousness may be experienced; this might also be felt by an attentive witness or audience. These states can involve changes to the sense of space and time; the sense of body boundaries might expand or dissolve; the surrounding air might take on qualities of light, colour, substance, expansion or motion; a mover might intuitively receive information from others in the space that cannot be known through the familiar senses. Mysterious happenings occur, empathic connections are felt, insight is revealed. For both the dancer and the Authentic Movement practitioner, these moments are gifts that we can only receive, the fruits of long hours and years of practice. They cannot be created or forced.

As Mary writes:

> *The image falls through the body, deeper and deeper, and then it gets light and spacious. It is present without effort.*
> (Fulkerson 1977: 93)

Through practise of the Discipline of Authentic Movement we might arrive in moments that are empty of thought, of content, of the need to find words and name our experience. Empty of personality and personal history, yet full of presence, of deep feeling and knowing. The paradox of being both full and empty cuts through separation of self from other and from the world we inhabit, so mover and witness might arrive in this place together – *empty mover, empty witness*, as Janet has named these places that we might, occasionally, in moments of *grace*, arrive at in our practice.[3] She writes:

> *At these times there is an experience of no edges, no boundaries. There is a sense of clarity, within and without, a feeling literally of no density, no obstruction, no place in the body through which light cannot move. In these situations the body becomes a vessel through which energy or light can pass unobstructed.* (Adler 1999b: 148)

> *For a witness this way of knowing can be manifest in an experience of clear seeing, seeing without the density of emotion or thought, increasingly at times without awareness of specific sensation. The witness can become empty in moments of direct experience. There are times when the mover knows when moving and the witness knows in witnessing that they are in a unitive state. Here the quality of experience for each is specific, imbued with timeless and infinite space.*
> (Adler 2002: 209)

In her beautiful poem – *Poem (the spirit likes to dress up)* (1986) – Mary Oliver speaks exquisitely to these ideas[4].

4: Somatic Movement, Somatic Imagination and Authentic Movement

In the last two chapters we looked at some principles of embodied awareness practice through the lens of three distinct but intrinsically related fields of practice: the somatic movement education and therapy approach of Body-Mind Centering; the somatic dance practice of Release Work; and Authentic Movement, in particular the approach named the Discipline of Authentic Movement. Within them there are differences in the ways of entering movement and developing conscious embodied awareness, sometimes just a subtle shift of attention; there are also many areas of overlap and connection between them. Whilst in practice they might sometimes weave together, each can be experienced as engendering a particular *mind*, a quality of attention and focus, which is distinct. In this chapter I would like to explore further some of the distinctions and meeting places, focusing on their shared areas of application that include education and healing, creativity and dance, and mystical practice.

Attention and Intention

> *Whenever one witnesses the state of the body, the interplay of thought and feeling, there is an intimation, however slight, of another current of energy. Through the simple act of attending, one initiates a new alignment of forces ... Opening to the force of attention evokes a sense of wholeness and equilibrium.* (Segal 1987)

Central to all embodiment practices is the act of paying attention, attending to sensations, feelings and the presence and movement of energy in the body. As Segal describes, this activates energy within the body-mind that can be clearly discerned by both one who is moving and another who might witness the movement. As attention awakens and deepens in the mover, the witness's own attention is deepened in resonance. But even before attention is awakened there is a choice to do this, an *intention to attend*.

When we 'remember' to pay attention to our bodily sensations and feelings we bring our mind and body, psyche and soma, into conscious relationship with each other. In the Discipline of Authentic Movement we seek to enter the movement with an open mind, with *naked attention*[1], receptive to whatever might be present or wanting to arise into consciousness in this moment. Something hitherto unconscious is knocking on the door of our awareness, seeking to become known, expressed and witnessed. We seek to keep on paying attention as each movement impulse, sensation, feeling, energetic flow, memory or thought comes into awareness and finds expression in movement, tracking the details of what we do and what we experience. Open attention might lead us into surprising places; we have entered the movement practice without a specific focus, intention or expectation, and impulses beyond our conscious control guide the unfolding of the process. The new, the unexpected, the mysterious are invited to arise into conscious awareness.

Yet there is intention at the beginning – I intend, and commit, to close my eyes, enter the movement space and listen inwardly, seeking to be as present to my inner self as I can be, waiting to see what might arise. There might be moments when a choice is made to go more deeply into whatever is arising or to step back from that edge because it does not feel safe enough, or because this is not the moment to enter that territory for some other reason. Moments of choice to follow this impulse or that one can arise in Authentic Movement. There is a play between will and surrender as attention deepens (Hartley 2015).

Paying attention to sensations, movement impulses and feelings allows us to keep returning to what is present, to what is wanting to emerge and become known. This approach has parallels in Buddhist meditation practices such as Zen, Dzogchen and Mahamudra, where naked attention is gradually cultivated as we develop the capacity to be with what is, rather than trying to hold onto, control or change our situation in some way. Through this practice we might eventually realise that we are not separate from all that meets our attention, as Nigel Wellings describes:

> [T]he witness itself will disappear entirely and instead of witnessing the sky, you are the sky; instead of touching the earth, you are the earth; instead of hearing the thunder, you are the thunder.
> (Wellings 2010: 138)

Some approaches to meditation begin with the intention to focus the mind on a chosen object until the mind is ready to settle within the body, into consciousness of the present moment, arriving into pure awareness and presence: the breath, a candle, a visualisation or a mantra can serve as an object of focused attention. The mind is invited to become one with the object of its focus. A somatic practice often starts in this way – with a focus, an intention to explore a specific movement pattern, or area of the body, or connection between bodily parts, or an image, for example. There are innumerable places to begin such an exploration.

Having said that, a somatic session can begin, even before an intentional focus enters, with a period of rest and relaxation, of stillness, inviting receptivity to what is present. A session often begins with a period of deep yielding into the support of the earth, allowing the body to gently release and soften so that space opens up inside. In Body-Mind Centering we might first attend to the presence of cells within the body (Bainbridge Cohen 2008; Hartley 1995); when the mind can settle there and we feel embodied within our cellular nature, we might have an experience of potent rest and stillness reminiscent of Mary's description of the stillness that is entered before a process of active visualisation in Release Work (Fulkerson 1977: 51).

Attentive and receptive listening to the body and what it needs might be followed by a process of intentional focus where we progress through stages of *touch and movement re-patterning*, as practised in Body-Mind Centering (Hartley 1995: 119). Areas of tension can be released, connections made and a core of inner strength and support may be contacted through the skilful application of the techniques and processes developed in this practice.

So we see that both approaches – beginning with an *intention* to focus in a certain way or beginning with open *attention* to whatever arises – weave together in practice. They might lead us into similar territory – the union (yoga) of body and mind, embodied presence. However, the place we start from and the path we take might create a subtly different taste, a view from a particular perspective.

In any movement discipline, from ballet to martial arts to yoga, the practitioner can practise from a place of the *body objectified* – How do I look? Am I performing well? Relating to our own body as 'other', as an object to be used, controlled and sometimes abused, rather than as the locus of subjective experience, is a common and problematic phenomenon in our modern times[2], though perhaps less so in traditional and indigenous cultures. A practitioner might be in dialogue with their body and its movement – tracking, guiding, intending or even forcing specific results. Or they may be at-one, present in the body, the movement, the moment. Then they are *fully embodied* – perceiving *from* or *through* the body. When authentic presence is wedded to skilful performance, attention and intention are in balance, and true mastery of the art can be achieved.

The Touch of Attention

Appropriate and caring physical touch is vital to an infant's wellbeing and healthy development, both physiologically and psychologically (Montagu 1986: Juhan 1987). The infant's sense of self is nurtured into being through touch; indeed, all through life we need to touch and be touched in order to maintain our physical and psychological integrity and sense of wellness (Hartley 2004). The healthy functioning of the nervous, endocrine and immune systems, and all the organs of the body, is deeply influenced by the experience of touch in infancy and throughout life.

I am writing this at the time of the coronavirus lockdowns when people all over the world are being forbidden to meet and to touch each other. But we are social animals. Our brains are designed to relate and be related to; touch and social engagement are as essential for our whole being as are food and water for our physical body. The question of how we sustain ourselves through long periods of touch deprivation, especially for those who are living alone, becomes a critical one at such a time.

The *touch of attention*, placed mindfully upon and within the body, can offer a nurturing alternative, a caress or embrace of awareness if you like – of course it is not the same as receiving another's physical touch and embodied presence, but mindful attention within the body can soothe, comfort, relax, connect and integrate. If we have received adequate touch in the past, whether as infants and children or as adults, our cells hold the memory of these experiences. This memory can be activated through the touch of our attention and some of the benefits might be felt again.

In the last chapter I mentioned how discovery of *empathy neurons* in the brain showed the mechanism by which, when seeing a movement in another person or imagining the movement in our own body, the same neural pathways are activated as if we were actually performing this movement. I imagine something similar to be occurring when awareness touches body with careful attention and an intention to soothe or heal or energise. Somatic work is ideally first experienced with the support of a skilled practitioner's touch; then the body remembers the sensations of receiving the touch and they can be recalled when practising alone. In this way, clients and students are empowered to embrace a personal practice that supports self-regulation and self-healing. (On my website I offer a few suggestions for somatic self-practice: *The Touch of Attention*[3])

Somatic Movement and the Potential to Heal

Somatic movement practice embraces a clear intention towards cultivating conscious awareness in the body, which fosters personal growth and healing; this can occur through an interweaving of *educational* and *therapeutic* approaches. Individual practitioners may focus their attention and intention more clearly towards one or the other but in somatic movement practice the distinction is rarely a clearly drawn line. We speak of *co-creation,* a shared journey of exploration, a dance between the practitioner and the student/client. An educational approach tends to be more practitioner-led; a therapeutic focus tends towards being client-led, though there will be much overlapping of approaches in a co-creative process. Both have the potential to educate, foster growth and heal through a shared creative exploration; each contains the other within it, just as Yin and Yang contain their opposite. When we touch the heart of a learning process there can be healing; when therapy touches deep into the core of the matter the whole self and sense of being can be re-educated and re-aligned from within.

The re-education of the body through somatic movement practice can lead to a greater sense of integration, balance and wholeness; healing and therapeutic change at both physical and psychological levels become possible as neuro-physiological changes occur. Somatic movement education depends very much on the skill and expertise of the practitioner who informs, guides, encourages or invites the client or student.

When the intention is specifically towards therapeutic aims, the process is clearly one of co-creation; it is the quality of *relationship* between the client and practitioner that enables the deepest change and healing to take place, enabled by the skill, sensitivity and responsiveness of the practitioner. Together they explore what lies beneath the symptoms, what might be trying to gain attention so that it can be brought into awareness, processed in the crucible of the therapeutic relationship, and move towards resolution: an inner struggle or tension that has not yet been acknowledged, deep feelings that have not been given expression, a part of the personality that has never been allowed to live fully. The psyche is reflected very precisely in the soma; somatic symptoms may have underlying psychological causes as well as sometimes causing or deepening emotional and psychological symptoms. This interplay is a constant fact of embodied life.

Working with Pain in the Body

Mary Starks Whitehouse, originator of the field of practice now known as Authentic Movement, wrote about movement that is functional: "For most people, the tempo and pattern of all physical movement is habit formed, automatic and, above all, organized toward a utilitarian end, toward an objective or goal." (Starks Whitehouse 1963: 52) This can include the quest to find comfort and ease pain in the body.

Physical tension, discomfort and pain are symptoms we are all familiar with and might be what bring a client or student to somatic movement sessions. Often, and understandably, the wish is to have something done to them so that the pain will go away. Sometimes this can be achieved with the skilful application of touch and movement interventions but often we need to explore deeper to contact the hidden source of the pain.

A somatic movement approach that embraces the psychological dimension of somatic experience can support such explorations (Hartley 2004; Aposhyan 2004), enquiring into the underlying emotional and psychological patterns that might be causing the symptoms. Authentic Movement also offers an approach to this (Pallaro 2007).

When intentions to achieve specific goals, including the easing of pain, can be suspended, then movement that is a spontaneous expression of the self can unfold. Starks Whitehouse described the latter as "'authentic' - it could be recognized as genuine, belonging to that person", which she came to view as the opposite of 'invisible', parts of the self where there has been lack of awareness. Both conscious and unconscious material informs the movement: "I move and I am moved." (Starks Whitehouse 1979: 81-2) Like image, which can serve as a bridge between these two realms, spontaneous authentic movement speaks of a truth which reaches beyond that which our consciousness alone can grasp.

I sometimes witness and hear a mover speak about their attempts to ease pain or physical discomfort – shifting, stretching, massaging the body to this end. This might come within the realm that Whitehouse referred to as functional movement, as might a remedial approach to somatics where the intention is to relieve symptoms and generally improve the condition and functioning of the body. Of course, there is a very real need and a valued place for this approach; often it is where we begin. Within the Discipline of Authentic Movement it is welcomed when done with conscious awareness. We can track these processes and connect to our self more deeply, knowing that there is pain and there are these movements we make to try to ease the pain. The body appreciates the kind attention, and the quality of our own touch might connect us to feelings of tenderness, self-care and love, or open us to memories of a gentle caress from a parent when we were very young and hurting, for example. The actions we make to soothe the aches and pains may eventually open us to a new path of exploration, beyond this immediate focus, when we attend with care and open awareness.

We can also enter more fully into the wounded place, the pain or discomfort, feel into its presence within us, its shape, movement, intensity. Allowing the sensations of pain to guide us, we follow the path that opens up, deepening to whatever lies within, beneath or beyond the distressing symptom. Sometimes tears of pain and frustration need to be shed and relief from the pain can often be found through this; the physical pain might be a manifestation of emotional pain and grief that needs to be expressed. We listen deeply and surrender to pain's message, inviting insight, guidance and deeper understanding of where we are right now and what we need in order to take our next steps.

Another way might be to ask – What else is there? Can I sense anything besides the pain in my body? What might lie beneath or alongside the sensations of pain and discomfort? By being with these questions with naked attention and curiosity, particularly in the case of chronic and pervasive pain, we can be opened to the underlying flow of impulses that take us deeper into our process. Here we might access what has been unconscious and calling for attention through the symptom. By allowing a spontaneous flow of movement to emerge, we come closer to the source of what is true for us in this moment. Sometimes the pain simply disappears: by not giving attention to it we have allowed deeper impulses from not-yet-conscious layers of our being to guide the movement and a source of wellbeing to be contacted; or a blocked process, which might have been the source of the pain, has been able to unfold, find expression and come to resolution.

At times the movement we make to explore, ease or work around our pain can itself become an opening into a surprising new movement pathway, evoking sensations, feelings and energetic phenomena that take us beyond the limits of the painful physical body. Mystery can be touched in such moments as suffering opens us to other realms of experience. As Trebbe Johnson writes, beauty can be discovered in the wounded places, both our own and those of the natural world:

> *The natural world, by virtue of its inclusivity, shows over and over that there is room for all phases and, hence, for all human reactions to those phases. When you see beauty in a wounded place, it is your own willingness to be seized by the anomaly that begins to shift your response to the nonbeautiful out of which it springs. And the more you allow the possibility, even the expectation, of beauty in a wounded place, the more susceptible you become to beauty in the bruised core of the human as well.* (Johnson 2018: 118)

Somatic Imagination and Dance-Making

The field of Somatic Dance emerged through dancers who also practised somatic movement or had trained in somatic dance practices such as Release Work, bringing deepened inner focus, the re-education of movement patterns and the fullness of conscious embodiment to their dance. A shift of attention can lead a somatic movement exploration towards creative exploration rather than educational or therapeutic aims. Mary's work is one example: a somatic approach to movement that invites balance, alignment, easeful and efficient use of the body, and opens into the art of dance-making. Her colleagues and mentors, including Marsha Palludan, Nancy Topf and Joan Skinner, all contributed to the development of this emerging field of dance.

I learnt from Mary what I have come to think of as *somatic imagination*. In a Release class, simple and known movement sequences – standing, walking, running, curving down, crawling, rolling, sitting, turning, unrolling to stand – might arise in a spontaneous flow as the image in the body evokes movement. As the dancer becomes at-one with the image, becomes the image, as Mary describes, the body and the imagination are no longer separate. Imagination is an expression of soma. Spontaneous movement is sourced in the felt-sense of the created then released image that now lives in and works through the body

– a map for new sensations which engender new ways of moving. The creation of new movement becomes endless.

I see this as different but intricately related to the practice of *embodied imagination*, as described by Jill Hayes (2007) and others, where images are given form through symbolic expression in dance movement. Many practitioners of Authentic Movement take this approach, sourced in the Jungian-influenced approach that Mary Starks Whitehouse introduced as "active imagination in movement" (Starks Whitehouse 1979: 84). In practice, somatic imagination and embodied imagination might interweave, but I see them as distinct processes.

Somatic imagination releases movement into expression without the intermediary of mental imaging. Dance is created spontaneously, sourced in the body. The dance holds the information that informed the image and it also arises as unique and idiosyncratic gestures and movements. The dancer plays with these arising gestures, develops and amplifies them. Something totally new might emerge. The dancer's internal world is made visible through the dance. She witnesses what is arising and also brings in an element of intention as she shapes the movement towards artistic ends. A spontaneous choreography. Attention and intention meet as the play unfolds.

The process of somatic imagination is one of 'coming into form'. We play through movement until form clarifies. The form may be a known pattern, such as one of the infant movement patterns (Bainbridge Cohen 1993, 2018; Hartley 1995) – for example, homolateral crawling or rolling through an integrated spine. Or it might be a unique and idiosyncratic gesture or movement sequence that becomes part of a dance. Psychologist Daniel Stern described four 'senses of self' that arise as an infant develops and also continue to endlessly arise throughout our lives: the sense of an emergent self, a core self, a subjective self and a verbal self. When we play with the *emerging of form* until recognisable movement patterns crystallise, or imaginative sequences that become part of a dance take shape, we are re-embodying the *sense of an emergent self* (Stern 1985: Ch 3), a process of coming-into-being. As the movement finds clear form and expression, the *sense of a core self* integrates. Whether we practice towards educational, therapeutic or creative ends, an affirming of our sense of core self can be experienced and celebrated each time we cycle through this process.

Interweaving somatic movement, somatic imagination and Authentic Movement

- ➢ *I begin today with a slow and gentle somatic movement sequence to warm-up and warm-in.*

- ➢ *Then I come to rest and focus on the Figure-of-Eight image – down the back and up the front of the body, up the back of the head and softening down over the face.*

- ➢ *I surrender to the movement the image invites, rolling with ease across the floor, limbs responding fluidly and creatively as somatic imagination is awakened.*

- ➢ *Now and then, amidst the free flow of movement, familiar developmental patterns emerge – navel radiation, homolateral yield and push, spinal reach. Listening to what my body needs, the sensations it offers to my awareness, it becomes possible to make choices to further clarify or develop these patterns.*

- ➢ *I make a choice to explore other simple movements, as in a Release class – sit, turn, crawl, unfold, stand, walk, curve down, crawl, sit, turn, roll. I find ease and a simple pleasure in this sequence.*

- ➢ *I can elaborate, draw out, play with subtle articulations that arise spontaneously within the sequence of movements. I create new combinations of gesture; new tones of expression emerge; somatic imagination evokes changing dynamics and idiosyncratic expressions that contain the original image as a support for everything that is within me and part of me.*

- ➢ *I arrive at one moment, lying on my back, and sense a change of attention. I am entering what I feel to be a process of Authentic Movement. Movement slows down and the quality of attention deepens and expands towards a new level of my being. I become aware of subtler impulses and the sensation of energy in my body, which I feel differently to the sensations that come through the pathways of the physical senses. My awareness is still anchored in the physicality of my body but it has opened out to include more of what is moving within me and around me. Awareness of the call of Soul,[4] and the presence of Spirit moving through my body, is awakened. I am entering the unknown as movement continues to unfold.*

The Discipline of Authentic Movement as Mystical Practice

Authentic Movement has roots in the three areas of dance, healing and spiritual (or sacred or mystical) practice. All of these have informed the emergence and development of the practice and Discipline, and find expression within it. All were present in Mary Starks Whitehouse's original explorations and continue to evolve in the work of practitioners today.

Healing

As mentioned above, healing on a physical level might come about, even without intentional intervention. Psychological healing is very much a part of the journey a mover embarks upon when they commit to entering the movement circle, again and again, often over many years, inviting unconscious material to arise, find expression, be witnessed by another and thus become known and integrated into consciousness. Connection to our inner self deepens and we become more whole, more fully who we truly are, through ongoing practice.

Dance

Sometimes movements arise spontaneously in an Authentic Movement session that are felt to have the quality of *dance*. The dance might be a personal expression of how the mover feels in the moment. Or it could be a spontaneous embodying of a cultural dance form that might or might not be previously known to the mover; I have witnessed in students the movements of classical Indian dance, Eastern European circle dances, as well as T'ai Chi sequences and other forms that are shared cultural expressions arising spontaneously out of the collective unconscious in that moment.

A dancer might also use Authentic Movement to source material for dance-making. Her inner witness is attentive to moments when a new pathway of movement opens up; she might track the sequence and return to it later, distilling material for the dance. Or, in the moment, she might make a choice to welcome somatic imagination and play with the gestures arising, shaping them with choreographic intent. Some have developed improvised dance performance based in Authentic Movement (Davis 2007).

Mystical Practice

In the Discipline of Authentic Movement, as developed and taught by Janet Adler, there is a recognition that there come times when we no longer need to keep unfolding the narratives of our personal history in order to deepen and enrich Soul and heal our psyche. We choose not to be led into choreographic concerns about how the movement might be shaped artistically. A time comes when everything that is extraneous to the direct experience of the moment can drop away and we are left empty, present with just what is. Authentic Movement becomes a mystical, or spiritual discipline, a path of connection to the Sacred.

In this way of working there is heightened awareness of all aspects of experience: the intricate details of the movement, gesture, sound, or stillness; the sensations we experience and the quality or movement of energy; emotional feelings, whether they are loud and demanding of attention or the subtlest hint of a feeling; the quality of the space around us; perhaps the energy of others in the room, or the environment around us, enter awareness. Staying present to what is, we do not need to interpret or find meaning in the experience, though insight might naturally arise.

In the time after moving, when we recall our experience and share with one or more witnesses, both mover and witness seek to open to deeper and more expansive layers, unfolding the moment in all its richness and fullness. We do not skip over this process with an easy labelling, which sometimes an image or metaphor can be, but keep asking – What else do I know about this moment?

In Vajrayana Buddhism we are told that every single moment can be an opening to awakened mind. Awakening is an ever-present potential and if we could just pay attention and let go, in the right balance, we might be graced with *Glimpses of Abhidharma* (Chogyam Trungpa 1975). Mostly, of course, we are not able to do this; it is not as easy for us as it sounds, but meditation practice supports us to prepare for glimpses of the true nature of reality. In the Discipline of Authentic Movement we take each moment of movement practice as such an invitation, an opening into direct experience of Spirit, the numinous, awakened mind. Keeping our awareness clearly grounded in the body, we can open to the potential for an embodied, immanent spirituality to become known.

Genuine readiness to practise in this way will come, for most people, after many years of moving and being witnessed; gradually we develop the capacity to stay present as personal and collective material arises into consciousness and can be integrated. We clear the density of our personal history as we develop embodied awareness; this prepares us for those moments when we can let go of our stories about past and future and simply be present with all that is, right now. Being embodied, a mover has learnt to contain and express both emotional and energetic charge, and can more safely enter the territory of mystical practice.

In this way of practising, attention focuses towards the subtle movement of energy in the body and a quality of sensation that seems to exist parallel to the physical sensations we are more accustomed to noticing. We might sense the energy body and its own realm of subtle sensation in such moments. Stepping into this realm of practice, allowing ourselves to be moved by forces that arise from neither our personal unconscious nor what we understand to be the collective unconscious, we transition from the work of psychological healing and *soul-making*, towards a *spiritual discipline*.

In my own practice these moments usually involve a slowing down and stilling; movement within the stillness and stillness within movement is palpable. As the moment empties of personal content, it is full with expanded awareness, feeling and the experience of pure energy, of Spirit moving through and around me. For others, these moments might come with abandonment to movement that is fast, energetic and vibrant.

Moving from image to developmental pattern to energetic phenomenon

> ➤ I am lying on my back, exploring the image from Release Work of my palms and the soles of my feet holding soft balls, and the space under my toes too. Somatic imagination awakens subtle articulations; intricate dances begin in my hands and feet. Imagination in motion.

> ➤ My awareness opens to many somatic possibilities: I can choose to focus on the skin of my palms and soles touching the air, the sensation of this; I can allow the air that touches my hands and feet to initiate movement in my body; or attend to the stretch and contraction of muscles, joints moving, organs supporting, nerve pathways giving soft focus and direction; I can focus on the Navel Radiation pattern[5],

allowing the play of opening and closing my body, the dance of all the limbs with the centre of the body. All of this is informed by Body-Mind Centering approaches to embodiment and is a familiar language for me.

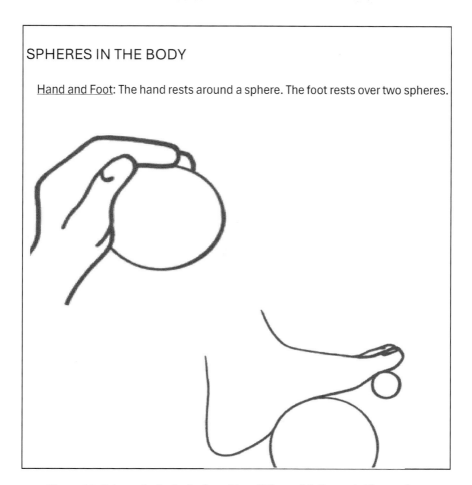

Figure 4.1: Spheres in the Body, from Mary O'Donnell Fulkerson's Theatre Papers

> *I am led more fully into the Navel Radiation pattern. At some point I am stilled, fully present within the experience of floating in the womb. I am right there – a body memory, clear and lucid, light filled in that moment. I am lying on my left side, my right arm and left hand softly reaching upwards. They are following the path of the umbilical cord*

towards the source of nourishment, of life – all life sourced in the placenta for the growing foetus. I float, feel peace, pleasure, wonder at the miracle of re-membering this experience before birth. I can stay with this embodied memory. Or –

- *I can let go of this focus and simply attend to what is happening within me in this moment. My awareness shifts into my energy body as I open into naked attention to all I can know about this moment. Letting go of all images, stories, interpretations, associations and memories, I arrive in embodied presence – just this, no more. Lying on the Earth, on my left side, my head easily lifted off the floor, supported by the flow of energy through my spine. My spine extends and arcs gently, my right arm extends into the space above – light, suspended, effortlessly held there. It reaches upwards and into the space which opens and expands around me. I feel totally supported and my body is at ease. I am empty of substance, pure energy. I could stay here forever – there is no need to move on, nowhere to go. I feel totally at peace.*

Body as Sacred Vessel – Body as Prayer – Body as Offering

The idea of the body as a sacred vessel through which Spirit, the sacred energies of the universe, the breath of life might flow and transform is not new. From the ecstatic dance of the shaman, the tribal dances of Africa, the postures of yoga or the flowing movements of T'ai Chi Chu'an, the sacred dances of India and Bali, the whirling of the Dervish or the circle dances of Eastern Europe – there are many ways in which people have strengthened, transformed, healed and expressed their sense of connection to Spirit, community and the natural world through the body.

Through the practice of the Discipline of Authentic Movement a mover may, at times, arrive in a place where they are opened to that which is greater than their personal self. Empty of personal story in that moment, the body becomes a sacred vessel for Spirit to move, and move through. Rather than through known and learnt forms, such as those named above, gestures arrive through an improvised journey into the unknown, carried by concentrated attention to what is present in the moment.

At times I experience moments of opening to a deeper sense of connection to Spirit and the Earth I am a part of, and my body becomes a prayer and an offering. Perhaps because our fragile world is so in need of help and healing right now, these moments arrive and become known in me like this. My body is an empty vessel, a wordless prayer which I offer up.

Authentic Movement practice (March 2020)

> - *As I step into the space, the palms of my hands want to feel the touch of the Earth. I come down, kneel, place my hands on the ground. My head slowly bows down until my forehead also touches the ground.*
>
> - *My hands begin rhythmically reaching out along the floor in front of me, with palms facing upwards and open; then drawing back in towards me. Offering and receiving. I become prayer. I feel humbled.*
>
> *I am filled with the magnitude of what is happening to humanity, the suffering and death; and alongside it the strength, generosity and compassion of the human Spirit. We need help.*
>
> *I feel the gathering of benign and healing energies surrounding the Earth like a crown, a corona of light, and I am humbled. I see this halo of light encircling the whole Earth and feel profound gratitude and awe.*
>
> - *Now I rise up, still kneeling. Spine and neck open and arch; face, throat, chest and belly are opened.*
>
> - *I move gently between the two – bowing to the Earth, opening to the Above.*
>
> *As I rise, I am drawing out a trail of hair between my fingers – it keeps the connection of my forehead to the Earth as I rise up. A feeling of joy, of bliss enters me.*
>
> *Bowing down, I am filled with respect, humility, gratitude to Mother Earth.*

To quote Trebbe Johnson again:

> *For all of us who live in this astonishing, fragile world, the choice to love that world, expand compassion for the others who share it, gaze at what's frightening and unpleasant, and meet it all with as much beauty as we're capable of is a radically conscientious act. When the*

gesture that pushes beyond individual isolation and into the unknown is aimed not just at breaking through a wall but also at bearing an offering, then the real rebellion begins: a rebellion of beauty as activism. (Johnson 2018: 193)

I will return to some of the themes touched upon here in the last part of the book, but will end this section by inviting you to search out a beautiful poem by Martha Postlethwaite, 'Clearing' (available online), that spoke to me during the time when the pandemic was beginning to close down activity around the globe – the time when much of the human race was forced to slow down, stop, go inward, pay attention to our own bodies and the Earth body in new ways.

Part 2

Embodying Spirit

5: Embryological Beginnings

I have endlessly questioned the title of Part 2 – Embodying Spirit. Is it too grand an idea, too difficult to write about, even harder to prove, something to be experienced beyond the world of words? And the answer kept coming back – yes, to all of these questions. Yet the phrase would not leave me alone, so here I am, trying to give words and some kind of shape to something both tangible and ineffable at the same time – the body infused with Spirit; Spirit embodied, at home in and expressed through the physical matter of a body.

I hope the last chapters have given a taste of how embodied practices, such as somatic movement and dance, and Authentic Movement, might approach the question of body infused with Spirit; how experiences of embodied spirituality might arise through the practice of these disciplines. There are many ways to explore and, at times, weave together these distinct but related approaches, as examples in the last chapter hinted at. They can also be applied creatively to investigate further into the embodiment of Spirit through the arc of human development, from conception through to the end of life. In the following chapters the reader will be invited into an exploration of how Spirit becomes embodied through the embryological journey and beyond; some exercises which draw upon the embodied practices outlined will be offered for those wishing to get a firsthand taste of some of the processes described.

So, to enter the search for words and the shaping of an idea, I want to go back to the beginnings of a human life, to the miracle of conception and the growing of the embryo that will become a foetus, an infant, a child and eventually an adult. But even before this, I will add a few more words to what I clumsily tried to name in chapter one about the term *Spirit*. There is everything and nothing to say about it, so I will name only briefly that I mean something akin to a pure, universal consciousness, sometimes experienced as an energetic vibration, a life force, light, love, the numinous – an invisible Source that flows through the Universe, the Earth and each of us who dwells here, creating diverse and sentient forms of life. In this view, all life forms are sentient – a blade of grass or a rock as much as a human being. I will return to this theme in later chapters, but for now, back to the embryo.

There are two perspectives on how consciousness and matter come together during embryonic development. One, described in brilliantly intricate detail by anatomist Erich Blechschmidt (2004) and in a different context by psychoanalyst Frances Mott (1959), sees matter and the physical laws of evolution as primary: out of the movements that arise during development of the embryo – dependent on the laws of nature, the physical forces that act upon matter – consciousness and a sense of self gradually evolve. The other perspective holds that pure consciousness or Spirit pre-exists the coming-into-being of a new life and becomes embedded in matter through the dance of conception and the growth of the developing embryo. Spiritual and religious perspectives, including Buddhism, which is one I have studied and practised a little, hold this view. Rupert Sheldrake offered a radical understanding when he described the *morphogenetic field* (1982). And embryologist Jaap van der Wal gives us a contemporary view of the process from a phenomenological as well as anatomical perspective (van der Wal online); he describes how the *gestures* the embryo makes as it grows into form show us the process of Spirit entering matter and shaping the physical expression of a new being. Our development is *in-formed* by Spirit. And with the evolving of physical form, psychological and spiritual potentials can unfold.

I like to think there is an interweaving of these two approaches, the coming together of which leads to the miracle of new life.

Van der Wal invites us to enter into the gestures of the embryo, to embody them, in order to experience something of what these gestures tell us about the embodiment of Spirit. The practices of Body-Mind Centering, Authentic Movement and Somatic Imagination are excellent vehicles for such embodied explorations.

Movement is Life

All living forms move as an expression of the life force that flows through them. Atoms and particles dance, they separate and come together, forming molecules. Molecules combine to form cells. Cells form complex living creatures and plants. All are alive, moving. Even the ground we stand on, the granite rock of the Earth, moves, slowly, defining time itself as she spins through space in her daily and seasonal cycles – a dance with sun, moon, stars and the space she revolves within, inspiring and expiring, renewing and recycling every form of life that inhabits her through these infinitely repeating motions. Earth breathes, following her own rhythms.

A human being comes into existence through specific movement sequences that are shared with a multitude of other life forms. Two cells meet and join together to form a new life, at first just one single cell that breathes, pulsing in a dance of expanding and condensing form, as the breath of life moves through and animates it. Just as the Earth herself breathes. Like the Earth, the fertilised cell takes the form of a perfect sphere containing all that it will become within its outer membrane.

The Dance of Conception – Feminine and Masculine

Nothing that we will become, create or experience has not already been experienced and expressed, in some embryonic form, during the process of embryological development. The embryo contains the plan and the potential for all that will later unfold; I hope this will become clearer as we go on. By exploring the movement journey of the developing embryo, we can discover many truths about ourselves as human beings and the roots of our being-in-relationship with others and the world we live in.[1]

Van der Wal speaks of the universal truth of the creation of something new when two polar opposites come together. When the polarities do not meet, but remain separated and out of relationship with each other, they will eventually die, physically, psychologically or metaphorically.

The *ovum* (egg cell) and *sperm* cell that must come together for a new life to begin are polar opposites:

The ovum takes the form of a sphere, a very stable structure; it is carried by surrounding currents and moves slowly through rotational motions; it is the only cell of the human body that is visible to the eye, having a large cytoplasmic body; usually just one ovum is released each month from the ovary of a woman during her menstruating years; it has a long lifespan, originating in the ovary of the mother when she was still in the womb of her own mother. The ovum connects us to our maternal lineage in a deep and intimate way, and to the principle of the Feminine and ancient wisdom: the seed of *you* was present in your grandmother's body before your mother was even born.

The characteristics of the sperm are the opposite of this: the sperm is tiny and linear in form, with a long tail to aid movement, a small 'backpack' of nutrients for the journey and a head which contains the cell's genetic material and vital organs for energy production, but little else; it moves in a primarily linear, directional way, having a purpose and intention, a goal to reach; the sperm cell is short-lived and will die or be reabsorbed back into the body if it does not fertilise an egg cell; millions of them are produced with each ejaculation. In the sperm cell we find the essence of the Masculine principle and the impulse to seek, to challenge and achieve.

In naming Feminine and Masculine principles here, I intend meanings related to archetypal essence and not gender identity, which is of quite a different order. I hope the reader can follow this convention of naming, and appreciate the biological expressions that underlie the terms without feeling the diversity of gender identity is limited by them. Each of us contains all potentials within us, in our own unique balance.

The journey of the ovum towards conception is a release from the ovary that has been home for years, decades even, then a path of descent down the fallopian tube towards the womb, a potential new home. This lays down a map for the initiatory journey of descent that women, and the Feminine in all of us, will undertake at those times when a passage must be crossed, our sense of self and a vital connection to life needs to be renewed or restored, and a new stage of life or way of being in the world calls us. Loss, illness, depression or depth initiatory practices might herald such a journey (Hartley 2001).

For the sperm cell, the initiatory journey begins with a dynamic release in ejaculation and involves a quest, the archetypal hero's journey where obstacles must be overcome, mountains climbed, rivers crossed, enemies defeated or outwitted and challenges met with courage in order to claim the prize of deepened connection to the Source of life, to wisdom and inner strength. The hero's journey celebrates the essential qualities and powers of the Masculine that are developed during the initiatory quest, whilst in pursuit of deeper connection with the Feminine within (Campbell 1988; Whitmont 1982).

Both ovum and sperm are 'birthed' from their respective first home. This is one of several mini-births that will take place during the process of conception and implantation, when a new home is found in which to nurture the development of new life. In our adult lives we sometimes find that a change of place is needed after a process of deep inner change, as our renewed sense of self might require fresh soil in which to grow.

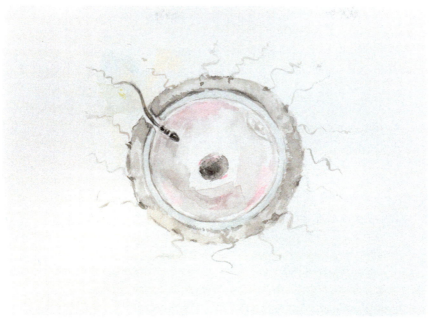

Figure 5.1: Dance of Conception – Ovum and Sperm (day 0, the beginning). Artist: Raima Drąsutytė

When the two cells come together, following a heroic journey on the sperm's part and an opening from the ovum's outer membrane, then a new life is about to come into being. The head of the successful sperm penetrates the ovum's outer membrane, as she briefly opens to receive him then seals the rupture to prevent others from entering. She appears to 'choose' the one she will allow to enter, chemical messengers softening the membrane at the place of contact. She is not a passive recipient or penetrated 'victim' in this act, but expresses agency, being both active and receptive. The egg now contains the nuclei of the two cells; they fuse in a dance that surely must be likened to an exotic embryonic ritual of courtship and love-making:

> *Through some force that is not understood, the egg's protoplasm starts to shimmy, violently. The nuclei of sperm and egg sidle towards each other, enlarge, and shed their protective membranes.*
> (Tsiaris & Werth 2002: 50)

They unite to form one nucleus that contains the genetic material of both mother and father; the combination of genes is totally unique for each fertilised cell (with the exception of 'identical' twins). From the very beginning of life, the archetypal principles of Mother and Father are within us, the very essence of us.

The fertilised cell, now called a *zygote*, is contained within a translucent protective sheath called the *zona pellucida*, and is surrounded by a halo of nutritional cells, the *corona radiata*. The zygote contains all that will be needed to guide the development of the new being. Of course, nourishment of many kinds will be required along the way, but all the information for the unfolding of potentials is held within the cell's DNA. Embryonic development, indeed life itself, is an invitation for these potentials to unfold.

How this unfolding is initiated is still one of the great mysteries of life. Despite several theories having been proposed, perhaps some mystery must be preserved as we approach the process of Spirit incarnating in matter. Not having concrete knowledge allows embodied experiencing, somatic imagination and direct intuitive knowing to enter. It allows each person to have their own unique experience and insight when exploring the gestures of conception and embryonic development through movement.

What happens next is a period of apparent rest as the zygote is carried on its journey down the fallopian tube. What is happening during this time? A time to rest, acknowledge, celebrate what has occurred, to 'fall in love', to invite Spirit to enter matter? This is a question we can take into our movement exploration:

Embodying Sperm and Ovum

- Find a clear space in which you can move safely, and stand for a moment with your eyes closed or your gaze lowered and softly focused. Feel your breath, feel your feet contacting the ground.

- Now begin to imagine that you are a sperm cell – small, very agile, quick, linear in form. You are on a mission as you begin to move, in any way you wish to, your long tail spiralling at speed to propel you forwards, darting past obstacles, finding the way through. You might feel you are in a race to get there first or that you are part of a team, all supporting each other so that one of you can reach the goal (sound familiar?).

- ➢ Feel the energy of this lively and focused movement challenge. Do you enjoy this goal-oriented way of moving? Is it a familiar way of being in life or do you prefer a slower, gentler, process-oriented approach?

- ➢ Gradually bring your movement to a pause and stand again for a moment, simply breathing and feeling your feet on the ground.

- ➢ Now imagine that you are the ovum – large, spherical, rolling slowly as you are released from the ovary and begin the long journey down the fallopian tube towards the inner sanctuary of the womb. You are helped by surrounding fluids and the wave-like motions of hair-like *cilla* that line the tube.

- ➢ As the group of successful sperm cells reach your place in the fallopian tube, they swim around you and set you in motion, rotating more fully and quickly on your axis. They are each trying to enter your protective membranes, releasing enzymes which are like a knock on the door, but *you* will choose the one to allow through.

- ➢ One sperm is 'invited' in, as the ovum's outer membrane briefly opens in response to its efforts and the chemical messengers it releases. The head of the sperm cell slips through, releasing its tail, and the membrane seals up again. The cell now contains the nuclei of both egg and sperm, which gradually 'shimmy' together and unite.

- ➢ Then you rest (for some hours), still being rolled down the fallopian tube, as if this momentous occasion must be acknowledged, celebrated, held in sacred time; perhaps it is a time to rest, to 'fall in love', to agree to continue the journey, to invite Spirit to enter matter. What might this moment mean for you?

- ➢ It is worth reflecting on the fact that you were, from your very first moment of conception, successful – the one who found the right path and won through, the one who was able to open and receive. You were a success story from the very start of life!

Inside – Outside

The fertilised cell, the zygote, is a being unto itself, floating freely in the fluid environment of the fallopian tube, not yet attached. It still has the form of the ovum, a perfect sphere, complete, containing a whole world within itself. It has an outer membrane, protected for now by the zona pellucida. Within the cell membrane is the fluid cytoplasmic body; it contains a nucleus and numerous organelles, which carry out the essential functions of cellular life.

Outside the cell membrane is another world – that of mother/other – also a fluid environment, vast and oceanic. In fact the salty fluids within and outside the cell membrane are microscopic drops of the Earth's ocean, captured at some point in the distant past; back in history's oceans, colonies of molecules were attracted to each other and joined together, forming membranes around collections of molecular chemical processes and creating the first organic cellular structures. The trillions of cells in our own bodies are much the same as these earliest evolutions of organic life on Earth.

The polarity of *inside-outside* is a dynamic that we will be challenged to deal with throughout our lives and it also begins right here, with the first breath of the newly fertilised cell as it draws into itself what it needs for nourishment and expels any waste that is no longer required. It will also send out chemical signals to other cells, to the cells of the mother's body, as its journey progresses.

Regulating our internal needs, both physiologically, emotionally, psychologically and spiritually, and learning to balance these in relationship to the needs of others and the requirements of the environment we are in, is an essential task. The infant and child must learn this complex balancing act as he grows, if he is to develop a healthy sense of self and relationships with others that are life-affirming, supportive and fulfilling. The task does not stop with early development – it is life-long. As our internal needs change, from moment to moment, and the responses and requirements from outside also constantly shift and change, we are endlessly in a process of learning the great balancing act of self-other, inside-outside. To become a well-balanced and integrated adult we will need some degree of mastery in this task of self-regulation. The original cell breathing is our first teacher.

One Becomes Many, Many Are One – contents and container

After some time has passed – twelve hours, a day or more – what can be seen externally is that the one cell, a perfect sphere, a whole world containing all that this new being will become, transforms into two cells. Inside the fertilised cell the nucleus has doubled its chromosomes, which have then separated into two nuclei, each containing the same genetic blueprint, the same potentials waiting to unfold, or not. The cytoplasm of the cell body separates into two areas, one around each nucleus, and membranes re-form around them to create two individual cells. This process continues for a few days, one cell differentiating into two sister cells through a repeated process of rupture and repair, until there are many. It is now called a *morula* (mulberry), as it pushes through the narrow passage from the fallopian tube into the open space of the womb – another of the 'births' that happen along the way, as if even before an embryo has formed, the challenge of birthing is being practised and prepared for.

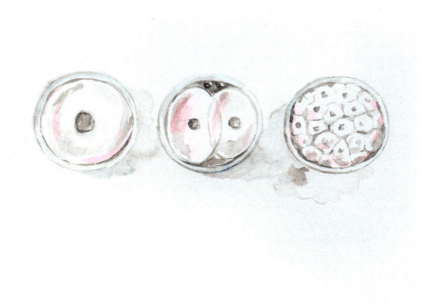

Figure 5.2: Cleavage – One becomes many (day 1-4)
Artist: Raima Drąsutytė

The cells, which until now have formed a cluster, all very much the same, begin to differentiate. Some cells gather together at one side of the sphere, forming the *inner cell mass*; others spread out to create a *containing membrane* just inside the zona pellucida, leaving a fluid-filled space within the centre. This new and transitory structure is called a *blastocyst*.

The inner cell mass will become the embryo. The outer layer will develop into a protective membrane to hold the embryo and foetus during gestation, and also contribute to the forming of a *placenta* to nourish its growth. This remarkable differentiation means that the embryo is both *content and container*. The membranous container is made of *self-tissue*, each of its cells having the same DNA as the cells which will become the embryo itself; the containing membrane will come into contact with the maternal tissue, but will not mix with it.

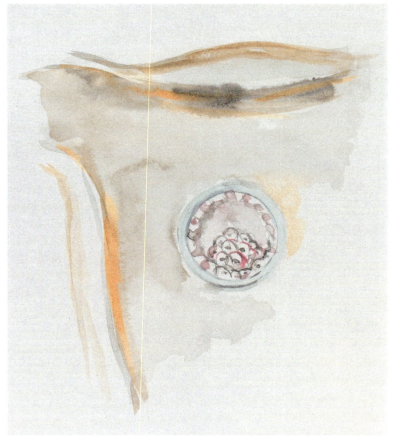

Figure 5.3: The Blastocyst – Inner cell mass and outer container (day 5-6)
Artist: Raima Drąsutytė

Contact will soon take place between this outer membrane of cells and the maternal tissues of the womb; this process demonstrates the seeds of personal boundaries, agency and relational engagement on the embryo's part. It can have profound implications for our later experience of being in the world and in relationship. We contribute to the holding of ourselves within the womb, active in the provision of both our own protection and nourishment; remembering this later in life can be a great resource for those whose womb experience has felt toxic or not safe enough.

I have worked with clients for whom the *knowledge* alone, that they create this layer of holding from their *own* cells, has been profoundly helpful. Knowing of this original distinction has enabled a process of differentiation from mother to begin, where this relationship has felt toxic and enmeshing. This might be further developed through somatic work that strengthens the sense of energetic boundaries and empowers the client in creating their own support and protection.

An Exploration – from one cell to many, becoming both contents and container

> ➢ You are invited to travel through this journey of differentiation, letting your somatic imagination play and shape your inner sensations and feelings into movement: imagine being one cell, floating through the fallopian tube, then differentiating again and again until you are many cells. The differentiations have a 'popping' appearance in microscopic views, as all the cells tend to double simultaneously in the first few days.

> ➢ As you become a more complex multi-celled body, feel how some of your cells spread out to form a membrane around you, containing the inner body of cells.

> ➢ Feel into this experience of being both the *contents* and the *container*. If you wish, allow your somatic imagination to lead you into dance, expressing what you are feeling in a creative way. Or you might let go of the focus and, allowing sensations, feelings and spontaneous movement impulses to guide you, deepen into Authentic Movement process.

➤ Afterwards, writing, drawing, or sharing your experience if you are exploring with others, can help to ground and integrate what comes up.

Coming into Relationship – self and other

Through all of this the blastocyst has been floating in the open space of the womb, searching for a place to implant, a home where it can put down roots and grow. Have you ever felt rootless and homeless, as if you cannot find the right place to live and have to keep moving house, searching for the good soil that will nurture you well? You might be re-enacting this earliest phase of life, some embryonic part of you unable to move on until the challenge of finding home is resolved, for this is what the blastocyst is doing. When it finds that place it will come close to the uterine wall and another miracle will occur.

The sphere of cells is still surrounded by the zona pellucida, which maintains the spherical shape and size of the original ovum. Imagine putting on a tight rubber wetsuit, then taking a deep breath in to get a feeling for the kind of pressure that might be felt here. The cells will feel the compression and eventually the need to break free will become strong enough for another 'birth' to occur. The urgent need to secure a source of nourishment will also be an impulse for what comes next.

Whether both mother and child are whole-heartedly ready to connect or not, if life is to continue implantation must occur. The zona pellucida breaks open and the inner cell mass *hatches*, just like a baby chick hatching out of its egg. This "allows it to expand and release the cells on its surface to interact with the outside." (Tsiaris & Werth: 57)

A chemical 'conversation' between blastocyst and uterine wall is now taking place, negotiating the possibility of making this place a home. The incarnating soul might experience the need to compromise, to make something akin to a 'contract' with mother in order that embedding in matter can happen safely. This *contract of the soul* is sometimes discovered as a psychological insight when people explore the stage of *implanting*. It might arise when there is a perceived unwillingness, ambivalence or vulnerability in the mother, and involves some compromise on the new being's part in order to be accepted, welcomed, supported and loved. For example, a message such as "I will be good / quiet / entertaining / helpful if you will love me", or "I will carry your pain so you don't reject or abandon me", might be discovered.

Such a 'promise' can become a script for the maternal bond, which can stay with a person for a lifetime if it is not brought into conscious awareness. Experiential therapy, such as somatic movement might offer, can invite these unconscious but powerful messages to surface.

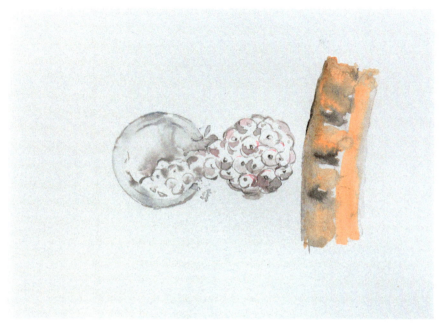

Figure 5.4: Hatching (day 7). Artist: Raima Drąsutytė

Willingness to open to connection and relationship, or remain as if still enclosed in the zona pellucida, can stay with us throughout our lives; or these impulses might appear and disappear at times, depending on how we feel, who we are with and the situation we are in. You can experiment, alone or with another:

Exploration of Hatching - coming into relationship

➢ If on your own, take a moment to imagine that you are wearing a tight rubber wetsuit, or something similar that you have a bodily memory of. Notice how you feel, how your breathing is, how ready you are to move, your willingness to meet others, engage in some activity.

- ➤ Then take a few deep breaths and imagine that the cells on the surface of your body expand and break out of the suit as it opens up. Again, notice how you feel, how your breathing is, how ready you are to move, your willingness to meet others, to engage in activity.

- ➤ Or you can try this with a partner. Sit facing each other and imagine you are wearing your tight suits. You might try having a conversation – about anything at all, just chatting or speaking about how you are feeling in the moment.

- ➤ Then both together, breathe and imagine freeing yourselves of the suit (hatching out). Continue your conversation. What changes? How do you feel and how does the interaction feel?

- ➤ You could also try the experiment, first with the 'suit' on, 1) through conversation, as above; 2) in silence, communicating only through eye contact; then 3) in silence, through movement and touch.

- ➤ Then imagine taking off the 'suit' and repeat these three ways of being in relationship and communication – through speech, eye contact, then movement and touch.

- ➤ Reflect on which way is most familiar and comfortable for you; when you might need to wear your 'suit'; when you most need to be free of it; how you release it if you need to; and what does all of this tell you about your relationship to incarnating, coming into earthly form and into relationship with others?

Now the outer layer of cells on the blastocyst's surface, the *trophoblast*, are free to come into direct contact with the mother, and enzymes are released that enable it to burrow into the surface layer of the inside of the uterine wall, the *endometrium*. This layer of maternal tissue will form the outer membrane of a three-layered protective capsule, the alchemical vessel that will contain the embryo and foetus. Here she will remain, completely enclosed, embedded within the endometrium, for the whole period of gestation. The pre-embryo has implanted.

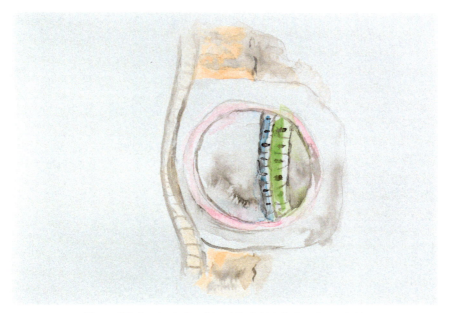

Figure 5.5: Implantation (day 10). Artist: Raima Drąsutytė

During the stages of conception and implantation many issues around incarnation – our readiness and willingness to commit to embedding in the world of matter – can be constellated. The quality of relationship between the mother and her child-to-be is seeded here; or perhaps it is constellated for the first time, as a 'decision' to incarnate was made even before conception took place and the seeds of their relationship may have already been present then. A sense that one or the other might not want the connection, or might be longing for it, or feeling ambivalent, can sometimes be 'remembered' when this stage is explored through conscious movement.

Continuing the exploration of implanting

> ➢ This exploration needs to be done with a partner and perhaps also a third person who will act as support and witness. One is the implanting pre-embryo; the other takes on the role of the womb-mother. The pre-embryo, with eyes closed and sitting or standing close to the womb-mother, takes time to feel into the possibility of making contact. The womb-mother sits or stands nearby, as open and receptive as possible whilst also feeling into her own willingness to connect.

- ➤ Take whatever time is needed to explore and feel into the journey of meeting. Both participants can allow their bodies to respond to whatever feelings, desires, needs and impulses might arise in relation to the potential of this first encounter.

- ➤ Notice which part of your body initiates contact, how this unfolds and how you are feeling.

- ➤ Listen to your body, allow it to move as it wishes, or remembers, for embodied memories might surface. Be as open as you can to what unfolds.

- ➤ Take time afterwards to reflect on and speak together about your experiences.

- ➤ When this feels complete, the roles can be reversed.

Bonding and Defence

Having found a protected home, a nest in which to grow, the next essential task is to secure a source of nourishment. Up to this point nutrients have been absorbed from the surrounding corona radiata and soon a *yolk sac* will form which will supply some nourishment for the next stages, but growth cannot continue for long without a reliable source of food and energy external to the embryo. This, of course, will come from the mother's body.

The encircling layer of cells that separated from the inner cell mass, and has engaged with the maternal tissue to form the container, will now also engage in securing nourishment. The two foundational principles which motivate our actions, *bonding and defence* – the desire to be close to that which we want, need, feel attracted to or identified with, and the wish to separate from or push away that which we do not want or feel threatened by – are both present in the functions of the outer membrane of cells, now called the *chorion*. These two impulses that will motivate our actions and choices throughout our lives are present at this earliest of moments. In Buddhist psychology their manifestations as *attachment* and *aversion* are seen as fundamental to our being in the world, and to the ways we create suffering for ourselves and others when they are not navigated with skill and awareness.

The *placenta*, the organ which will provide nourishment for the growing embryo and foetus, begins to form from the chorion. As noted, the chorion is a *self-structure*, evolved from the same original cell as the embryo itself; it is in intimate contact with the membrane of the uterine lining and together chorion (embryo) and endometrium (mother) contribute to the forming of the placenta. The placenta comes to maturity over a period of weeks (See *Figure 6.2*), but the chorion is engaged in drawing nutrients and oxygen from the maternal blood from the very beginning. Only once this has been established can the development of the embryo itself truly begin. As the placenta develops, reservoirs of maternal blood form within it; from this the nutrients and oxygen the embryo needs diffuse through the maternal and embryonic membranes and are pumped through vessels within the umbilical cord, to and from the embryo.

I feel the wisdom of this is profound. The need for a secure environment, a protected place with boundaries that have integrity as well as responsiveness to both inner and outer worlds is primary. Only then can the equally essential need for healthy sustenance be secured. In life, to live with integrity and wellbeing, not too vulnerable to the world around us and not too closed off from it either, we need boundaries that are firm, embracing, flexible, semi-permeable, in relationship and responsive to both our own needs and feelings and those of others. If boundaries are too rigid or too permeable, too thick or too thin, have gaps or tears or other damage, we will struggle in many ways and growth into full maturity will be hampered.

To develop the integration that we seek throughout our life's journey, to embrace our wholeness, clear and responsive boundaries are essential. This begins *in utero* with the quality of the protective membrane and all that it expresses for us. It is also reflected in the membranes of every cell in the body and in our skin, the interface of body with world. These membranes can yield information about the quality of our psychological boundaries when we listen to their condition, what they might lack and may need. Later we will explore the possibility of expanding, dissolving or releasing our sense of boundary, but first we need to clearly establish it.

It seems to me that the protective membrane which develops *in utero* will, after its physical existence ends with birth, continue to be present as a sensed *energetic skin,* embodying awareness of our personal space. We can sense and feel the presence of this energetic skin when we attend to the space around us that was once the place of the membranes in which we developed as an embryo and foetus. I will return later to this and other issues touched upon in this chapter, as dynamics that have their roots in embryological growth evolve throughout the life cycle.

6: Emerging into Form

Attention turns to the forming and growing of the embryo itself, now that a safe and nourishing environment has been created. *Support before movement* is a principle of Body-Mind Centering, and so it is for the embryo. Development is movement, a perpetual flow of motions and gestures which shape the new being into form. This movement can begin now that support has been established.

As mentioned earlier, psychologist Daniel Stern writes about the *sense of an emergent self* that precedes the coalescing of a *sense of core self*, which is the first necessary stage of psychological development after birth (Stern 1985). I would suggest that this process is already underway *in utero*, first in the embryonic forming of the foetus, with all its organ systems present, then in the multitude of preparations for birth and life beyond the womb. The emergent stage is one of process, where clear form is not yet apparent but is gradually emerging through many experiences that are not yet fully integrated; psychologically this means there is not yet an integrated sense of self, but a process of self-coming-into-being can be witnessed. The infant, until about two months old, is primarily in this emergent phase; then a distinct change can be perceived as a clear sense of the individual emerges. An infant will now look you directly in the eye and smile, and you will know that they are seeing you and responding as a person, a unique individual with a distinct core of beingness.

A precursor for this critical psychological development has already taken place within the physical forming of the embryo, as a process of endless shape-shifting, creating and dissolving of forms, folding, enfolding and unfolding takes place.

Growth is never linear but occurs in overlapping waves and spirals, yet some significant landmarks and stages can be identified amidst the complex flows of movement, thanks to special photographic techniques that have been developed (See Nilsson 1990; Tsiaris 2002; Blechshmidt 2004; van der Wal).

These emerging forms come about through the flows of fluids and cells – streaming, gushing, pulsing, migrating from one place within the embryo to another, gathering together and bulging here, stretching out there, circulating around the body or finding a location to stay awhile and grow into tissue. Cells and fluids in motion are the process of embryonic development.

In the pre-embryo, first the cells form into two parallel layers, which will become the front and back of the disc-shaped body. The cells of the front layer *(endoderm)* will contribute to the creation of the digestive tract, organs and glands. The cells in the back layer *(ectoderm)* will form the skin and nervous system, including nerves, sensory organs and brain. Then a third layer of cells will form between them *(mesoderm)*; this layer will eventually form muscles (including heart), bones, blood, lymph and connective tissues.

These three layers carry the life force, differentiated into *body* (mesoderm), *feelings* (endoderm) and *mind* (ectoderm) according to body psychotherapist David Boadella (1987). As adults we each come to organise these dynamics within our psyche in unique ways and their re-integration can be a focus for therapeutic work if they have become separated or imbalanced through trauma or adverse conditioning (Hartley 2004: 176). For example, one person might develop an overly mental approach to life, suppressing feelings and body awareness. Another might be too easily flooded with emotions and find it hard to express them in a clear way, or to contain them enough to reflect on what they are truly feeling. Yet another person might be driven by a need to be physically active, perhaps compulsively or competitively so, without the capacity to know healthy limits.

Some cells from the ectoderm and mesoderm spread out behind the body to form a fluid-filled sac, the *amnion*. Cells from the endoderm and mesoderm migrate out to form a *yolk sac* at the front of the embryonic disc, which provides some nutritional function and produces blood cells in the early stages until the liver, bone marrow and spleen develop and take over this function. Later, part of the yolk sac will be re-absorbed into the body and some of its cells will contribute to the forming of the reproductive organs.

For a while the embryonic disc is held between these two large fluid-filled sacs, like two giant cushions supporting it – the yolk sac (nutritional 'mother' function) at the front of the body and the amniotic sac (protective 'father' function) at the back. Between them a subtle flow of fluids passes in a slow rhythm, front to back, back to front, through a tiny space in the centre of the embryonic disc, so that the yolk and amniotic sacs alternately fill and empty just a little.

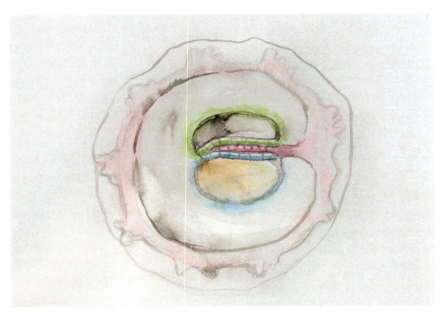

Figure 6.1: Three-layered embryonic disc held between amniotic and yolk sacs (week 3). Artist: Raima Drąsutytė

The rhythm of a subtle flexion and extension of the whole body is imprinted within the cells of the pre-embryo and becomes a foundation for the rhythm of opening and closing, extending and flexing, internally and externally rotating, which will underlie the rhythm of our journey through life. This rhythm seems to be a precursor to the *long tide* of the cerebrospinal rhythm, which is central to the balancing of the craniosacral fluid in Craniosacral Therapy (Kern 2001: 22) and the *autonomic nervous system rhythm* (Bainbridge Cohen 2008: 165). I am grateful to Bonnie for her research in this area, which inspired the following exploration:

Dance of the amniotic and yolk sacs

> ➤ Take a moment to imagine two large, membranous, fluid-filled sacs, one behind and one in front of you, completely supporting you and subtly filling and emptying in a slow rhythm, slower than your breathing, as fluid seeps between them. Take time to sense the subtle initiation of each phase of this rhythm – a subtle extension and opening out and a flexing, folding in towards centre. Wait until you can truly feel your own rhythm, allowing your whole body to slightly open out and then fold in as you feel moved by this rhythmic flow.

> Can you feel the support and balance the embodied memory of the yolk and amniotic sacs can give you?
> Inviting somatic imagination to awaken, you might allow a fluid, rhythmical dance of opening out and softening in to emerge. A dance of opening to meet the world and returning to self.

The growing embryo gradually curls into a deep C-shape, and the ectoderm layer at the back grows around the whole body surface, drawing the amnion with it to form the innermost layer of a now three-layered membranous container – the inner two layers are formed from self-structures (amnion and chorion) and the outer layer from the endometrium of the mother's womb (decidua capsularis). The shaping of organ systems within the embryo can now unfold.

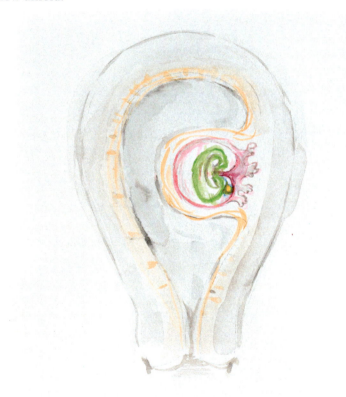

Figure 6.2: Three-layered membranous container and placenta (week 5).
Artist: Raima Drąsutytė

Bringing the Outside In

A meditation – inside, outside

- ➢ Sitting in a comfortable position, close your eyes and take a moment to follow the flow of your breath, in and out of your body. Allow your mind to settle and your body to release weight into the supporting surfaces of floor, chair or cushion.

- ➢ Become aware of what you sense and feel within your body, simply noticing, without holding on or pushing away, without having to change anything at all.

- ➢ Then expand your awareness into the space around you. Let your external senses open and notice what comes to you from outside.

- ➢ Take your attention wider – can your senses receive impressions from the environment outside the room? There might be sounds, changes of light, smells, currents of air if a window is open.

- ➢ Now imagine/remember the neighbourhood you are in and, extending your awareness to this outer environment, notice the impressions, the sounds, sights, smells that you receive from there.

- ➢ You can expand your awareness even further – to the town or city where you are, to the whole country, to the continent, the planet and beyond. Go as far as you feel able and comfortable. Receive the sensory, remembered and imagined impressions that come to you.

- ➢ Gradually begin to return, reversing the journey through each environment, until you arrive back in your own body. Sense and feel into yourself. How are you now? Has anything changed? What do you notice?

This simple experiment[1] invites us to explore the relationship between body and consciousness, and to recognise that consciousness, whilst being anchored in the body, can also extend far beyond it. As we expand our awareness then return to our self, bringing some of the 'outside' back in, we may feel changed in some way. We may even feel the presence of Spirit both within and beyond us.

This seems to be what the embryo does as it begins to develop. As we follow the gestures its emerging forms make, we see a process of involution taking place through each of the three embryonic cell layers – mesoderm, ectoderm, then endoderm: cells on the outer surface multiply and turn inwards to contribute to the formation of internal structures within the developing embryo. As we embody these gestures, we might get a taste of what they are showing us about the nature of becoming a human being, Spirit embodying in matter.

Heart

The inner cell mass, now shaped like a disc with a front, back and middle layer, is growing rapidly as cells continue to multiply. To support this growth, it will need a circulatory system to deliver nutrients to all the cells, those deep inside as well as those on the surface. Hence, the first organ to begin to function is the embryonic heart and it develops from the middle mesoderm layer of cells. It begins life as two connected tubes of primitive muscular tissue which, at only eighteen days old, have already begun to pulse. The heart is born. And in this first incarnation it lies at the surface of the embryo in the place which will eventually become the forehead. The embryonic heart looks up and out. This location also ensures that the blood supply will go first to the nearby developing brain.

Other developments (which we will come to in a moment) are causing the back body to bulge out so that the front body folds deeply. The head-end, which is growing rapidly, bows downwards as it is drawn towards the tail-end in a deep C-curve, and with this gesture the developing heart is brought down and in, to the centre of the chest. Here it finds its home, deep in the centre of the body, and gradually it will evolve into a fully formed heart with four chambers, a powerful spiralling muscle that will keep beating throughout a lifetime. We can imagine that in this gesture it draws in and down some of what it has opened to in its brief time of looking up and out from the head of the embryo. From the light and space of above, the heart descends into the density of matter.

Throughout our lives, balancing the needs and wisdom of head and heart are at the centre of many choices and challenges. The embryo shows us that heart and brain begin in intimate relationship, touching each other, with just a membrane between them, before the heart travels into the centre of the body. Here it can be felt to be an underlying support for the brain. A life's journey requires us to keep remembering this close bond between our thinking and feeling self.

An Exploration of the Descending Heart

I find it best to do this standing, but sitting is also possible.

- ➤ Take a moment to close your eyes, feel your feet (or sit-bones) resting on the ground and breathe. Let thoughts settle and awareness arrive in your body.

- ➤ You can imagine that your legs are an extension of your torso, like the distinctive long tail which is emerging at this embryonic stage; this can help you to feel that your whole body engages with the movement.

- ➤ Now imagine that your heart rests at the top of you, sitting at your forehead, opening up and outwards. Feel into this gesture, what it might be communicating, how it feels to allow your heart to be open to the space above. Let your body, or perhaps just your hands, express how you feel in this gesture, then follow the descending journey the heart will make. Let your hands imagine into this moment and express it creatively if you wish.

- ➤ Very slowly the body curves forward, head and tail-feet moving towards each other, as the heart moves towards its place in the centre of the chest area. It is not physically possible for our adult body to complete this movement, but imagine and feel its potential. You might be activating a very old memory as you do this. Again, sense into how this feels for you, what does the embryo communicate through this gesture.

➤ You can repeat the movement as often as you wish, feeling into what it means for you, allowing your somatic imagination to dance you as you express the feeling; or there might come a moment when you are called to deepen into an Authentic Movement process, allowing whatever is present to move you.

➤ As this is happening in the embryo, the arm buds are starting to emerge from the sides of the chest area and they come to fold over the heart as it arrives in its central place. As this process completes, the embryo looks like a little Buddha – growing legs loosely crossed, hands folded over heart, chin resting on chest – drawing in what was outside and contemplating it.

➤ Come to rest. You might like to draw or write about your experience to express and anchor it in consciousness.

Nervous System

Whilst this is taking place, the cells at the back of the body, the ectoderm, are multiplying at a rapid rate. A functioning brain and nervous system will be needed in order to co-ordinate the development of all other physiological functions, and this is where it begins. Single cells throughout the growing body are continuously differentiating into two sister cells, doubling their chromosomes then separating into two more or less identical twins, just as the original fertilised cell did. One of the sister cells will continue the process of differentiating into two, while the second sister cell will now begin her journey towards a specific form, function and location in the body.

Much of the ectoderm layer will develop into skin, but many of its cells will become the nervous system. Groups of multiplying cells begin to form a bulge along the back body, then they involute along the length of what will become the spine and brain. Turning inwards from their external location, they form a tube inside the embryo, the *neural tube*, which separates from the outer skin-layer of cells. The primitive nervous system is born. The cells on the surface come back together to close the gap, the valley that formed along the length of the back, reintegrating the outer skin layer.

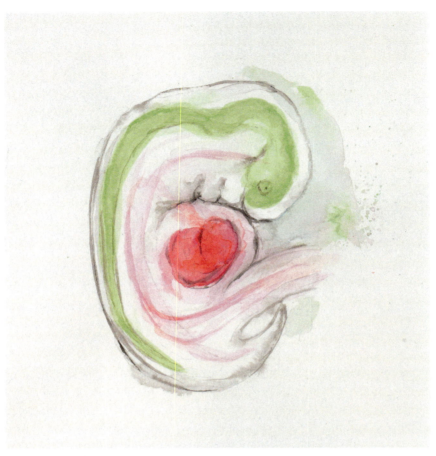

*Figure 6.3: Heart and nervous system – bringing the outside in (from week 5).
Artist: Raima Drąsutytė*

Although now separated from the skin, the nervous system will always be intimately connected with it because of their shared origin in the ectoderm. Deane Juhan has called the skin the outer surface of the brain, or the brain the innermost part of the skin (Juhan 1987: 35). Touch to the skin will always reach our deepest core. What we experience in our depths is revealed through our skin. We also rely on the sensitivity of our skin to know the world around us. Touch is essential for life, for growth of the nervous system and other essential organ systems; it enables us to meet and relate to the world outside of us in meaningful ways and it enables our inner world to be made visible in the outer world (Juhan 1987; Montagu 1986).

With a neural tube developing, the complexity of evolving a brain, nerve pathways and sensory organs can begin. From the neural tube, which will become the brain and spinal cord, fibres reach back towards the surface layer, meeting skin again, forming sensory organs within it and connecting them to the brain; a system of two-way communication and feedback begins to evolve.

The gesture that is the involution of cells that form the neural tube takes place through the motions of cells as they multiply and stream into place, each seeming to know just where to go, what it will become. This 'plan', described by Sheldrake as the *morphogenetic field* (1982), is one of the great mysteries of life. It appears that all cells, which begin with exactly the same DNA and more or less the same internal environment, take on specific form and function due to the locations they move into and the pressures they are under whilst moving into their place and being there. Blechshmidt writes about how muscle cells, for example, are subject to pulling and stretching, and this creates the long fibres which will have the capacity to contract, release and thus move body parts (2004: 145). Every other type of cell will be similarly informed by the pressures they experience; out of this, form and function will evolve.

Embodying the formation of the neural tube

- ➢ This exploration is best done with another person but you can also visualise, sense, feel and invite somatic imagination if exploring on your own.

- ➢ One partner can lie down, on their front if this is comfortable, or else on one side. The other will offer gentle touch to the whole length of the back surface, from the centre up to the head and down to the tail of the spine. The focus is an invitation to the cells to breathe, to expand and fill with breath. Breathing freely, imagine they can multiply and move with the flows of surrounding fluids. The quality of touch can offer this as an image and a potential.

- ➢ The person lying down imagines, senses and feels into this potential.

- ➢ Together both visualise the involution of cells along the length of the spine, the streaming of groups of cells inwards, from the body surface, to form a tube of cells along the whole length of the spinal cord and up into the brain area. It separates completely from the outer layer of cells, then the skin cells on the surface close over to 'seal' the valley that has opened up. This happens from the centre downwards and upwards, the head and tail ends being the last to close. The partner sitting can gently indicate these directions through their touch.

> Make sure that the closure is complete, especially at the head and tail ends, as leaving an opening here can give a 'spaced-out' feeling and allow energy to leak away.

> The one who has been receiving the touch might want to move, to explore the feeling of the gesture of the neural tube forming. The other can continue making supportive contact or sit back to witness the movement unfolding.

Digestive Tube

By the time it is four weeks old the embryo will have a heart beating in the centre of its chest, already pumping blood that carries oxygen and nutrients to all cells of the growing body. It will also have a rudimentary nervous system, with the brain in particular growing at an astonishing rate. The embryo and foetus will receive all of its nourishment from the mother through the placenta and umbilical cord; blood containing nutrients from the placenta is carried directly to the developing liver, where it is pre-filtered before being distributed to the brain and the rest of body. The embryo also needs to prepare a digestive system which can function after birth when the source of constant nourishment from the placenta will cease.

Out of the third layer of germinal cells, the endoderm, the digestive tract develops, first taking the form of a simple tube from mouth to anus. A space has opened up along the length of the front body, another way that the embryo brings within itself something of the space outside. Although sphincters will in time form at key locations along this tube, the digestive tract is essentially a space within the body that is open to the space outside. The lungs too, as they form, are open to the outside, so that the air inside of our lungs is always continuous with the air outside. After birth, and throughout our lives, we share this air-filled space with all beings.

As the embryo curves into a deep C-shape with the growth of cells in the back body, as described above, you can imagine that the front body becomes compressed. There is little space for the digestive tube, which lengthens as it grows. It 'spills out' into the umbilical cord and coils up alongside the blood vessels that reach between the embryo's navel and the placenta. It will continue to grow within the umbilical cord, outside the body, until around the ninth week when the now-foetus begins to straighten out of its C-curve shape; this allows the tube, now developed into the small intestines, to spiral back inside the body wall to arrive in its place, in the centre of the abdomen.

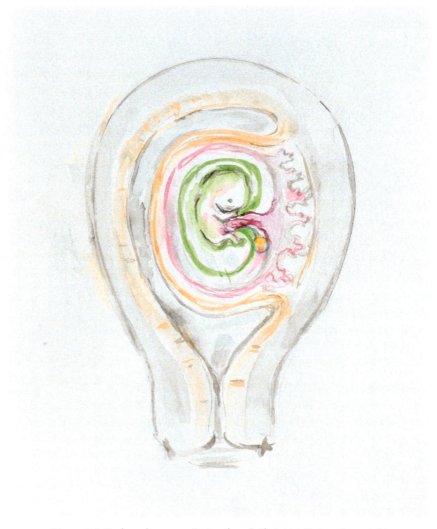

Figure 6.4: Embryo becomes Foetus (week 8). Artist: Raima Drąsutytė

The embryo has formed into a foetus by eight weeks, all of its organs present and ready for a period of growth and maturation. Soon after this, the eyelids have formed and will close for the next several months of foetal life. The ribs will also complete their development, meeting the sternum (breastbone) at the front of the chest to close the rib cage. It is as if the foetus now draws inwards to focus on the task of growing and maturing for the next five months, until ready to begin preparing for birth and the world beyond the womb.

Organic Origami

First the cluster of cells that was the blastocyst reached out to form protective and nutritive membranes to support the growing embryo; then groups of cells that were on the surface of the body turned inwards to form deep internal organ systems essential for life.

Many more developments have been taking place; lungs and respiratory system, reproductive organs, kidneys and bladder, spleen, lymphatic organs and vessels, endocrine glands – a complex process that has been likened to origami takes place, with groups of cells streaming, gathering, folding, unfolding, forming, dissolving and re-forming in another shape and location. The kidneys, for example, make a fascinating journey. They begin as two small structures near the area that will later become the shoulder blades. Then they dissolve, cells migrate down and re-form in the back of the pelvis, near the tail of the spine. They dissolve again to re-form in the back of the lumbar area, one on each side of the spine and just below the diaphragm, where they will remain. Taking some time to trace and sense into this journey can bring rest and grounding to the kidneys, organs which are often felt to carry stress and tiredness.

When there is disruption, trauma, stress, perhaps a lack of support for mother or embryo, some part of the embryo's energy system might become 'stuck' at that delicate stage of development, frozen in time. Such disruptions can manifest later in life as places that feel numb, disconnected or tense, for example; they can manifest in both the physiology and function of the body, in the organisation of the psyche, and in the capacity to stay connected to Spirit. Minor disturbances can be accommodated but sometimes more significant disorganisation can become embedded within the cells, tissues and nervous system, causing problems. By embodying the gestures of embryonic development, we might get a feel for the quality of energy and attention that was present at that stage and still lives within us as "the place of space", as Bonnie has called it (Bainbridge Cohen 2008: 163). Healing of primary disruptions becomes a possibility.

The mystery of involution and evolution, a series of gestures which express and integrate polarities of masculine and feminine, inner and outer, container and contents, self and other, front and back, left and right, up and down, all shape and re-shape the embryonic being until the foetus is formed. Providing no genetic variations have created a differently formed body (which of course does sometimes happen), the eight-week-old foetus will now contain all of its organ systems, tiny, not yet mature and fully functioning, but ready for the next phase of development.

An Exploration, a Dance

- ➢ You can explore and express some of these landmark moments creatively, following the gestures of opening out and drawing in; holding and being held; streaming, pulsing, gathering, releasing; folding and unfolding; shape-shifting as gestures emerge and dissolve in the process of coming into form.

- ➢ Go where you feel drawn and allow your somatic imagination to explore creatively. If you like, play some music which suggests these processes to you; this can be a support to moving freely. Or perhaps explore in a space enclosed by soft cushions and blankets to replicate the womb.

- ➢ Continue after the movement exploration to unfold and bear witness to your experiences in writing or drawing.

Unfolding to Verticality

If we could see the embryo and foetus's development as one continuous gesture, we would see a very slow rhythm of opening and closing over a period of weeks and months; this movement, like breathing, is a basic pulse of life. Beginning life as a perfect sphere, then a spherical cluster of cells, the pre-embryo then opens, flattens and lengthens out to form an elongated disc. As the embryo begins to grow it curls in around itself, head and tail almost touching, as it brings its heart into the centre and returns to the roundness of its first gesture. Gradually, as the neuromuscular system begins to develop, muscles along the back of the neck engage, lifting the head upright to bring the embryo into a vertical gesture, head aligning with spine in the familiar human posture.

The umbilical cord lengthens and the foetus moves away from the placenta; it turns to face the source of nourishment, now able to relate to mother for the first time as it finds space and a small measure of separation. In this essentially vertical alignment, the arms and legs are developing. Soon active movement becomes discernible and the tiny foetus has a great deal of freedom to 'dance' within the fluid filled space of the amniotic sac, supported, held, buoyed by the fluid environment rather like an astronaut floating in space. Scans have even revealed the young foetus performing somersaults in the womb.

The gesture of aligning through the vertical axis is almost uniquely human amongst mammals. Most animals move about on all fours most of the time, coming to vertical on occasions but returning to the earth when stability and speed are required. Van der Wal suggests that this gesture of verticality is an expression of the human alignment with both Heaven and Earth, an intimation of the potential for spiritual life that exists within each of us: the meeting of Heaven and Earth within the human body, with the heart at the centre, feet on the ground and head reaching into the sky above. He developed this idea from a phenomenological approach of embodying the gestures of the embryo; the question of the spiritual life of more-than-human life forms will be touched upon from other perspectives in Chapter 12.

It is in the gestures of the limbs that we can see this evolution most clearly. The anatomy of the human shoulder joint is quite different from that of so many of our four-legged friends. The limbs of most mammals move primarily in the sagittal plane, flexing and extending for forward movement; they offer no significant rotation, adduction or abduction. This gives stability, power and speed in running, but it means many of the gestures that humans can make are limited.

The complexity of the human shoulder joint allows us to open our arms wide to embrace; draw hands together in prayer or gratitude; move forwards and back to give direction and purpose, to offer and receive; reach upwards in longing or aspiration, or down to the earth in reverence and humility. The energy of the heart is intimately connected to the arms and hands, and the rainbow of gestures that flow from the heart are expressed through them. We can stand and walk, rooted to the Earth and the sky through our verticality and at the same time express a whole range of human feelings through our gesturing hands.

A four-legged creature walks with forelegs vertical, paws firmly in contact with the Earth. The heart is in direct contact and communication with the Earth. With each step the non-human animal renews and maintains a heart-Earth connection. An infant too, for a period of time, moves primarily in this relationship to the Earth. Try it – mindfully crawl on all fours, with awareness centred in your heart and the contact of your hands with the Earth. Can you feel how grounding this is and how intimate your connection with the Earth becomes? Do you feel the deep support for the heart, how being in this relationship can be a way of listening to the Earth, acknowledging that you are part of her, that your animal nature and Earth nature are the same? Can you also feel how different your connection with above and all around you is when your focus is down into the Earth and straight ahead?

The gesture of limbs perpendicular to the body is present in non-human animals *in utero*. Imagine spending all those months, held within the womb as you grow, with your four limbs placed out in front of you, bending and flexing a little as if running, but your hands unable to come in to caress your own face, unable to rest over your heart as if in prayer or reach up and out to explore and contact all dimensions of the womb-world around you. These gestures are seen in the human foetus, and when we embody them in somatic explorations we can feel into the meanings that they communicate – something about a deepening relationship to self, to other and to Spirit may be discerned.

As the foetus grows it eventually fills the whole space of the womb. In the last two months of gestation the space begins to feel tight and the restriction of space folds the foetus back into a curved form, limbs tucked in, head and tail reaching towards each other again in the familiar foetal position. The little one is preparing to birth: muscle and organ tone is stimulated by the pressure from the muscular walls of the womb, so that the power needed to birth can develop. The protected space of the womb might begin to feel more like a prison and the need to emerge from it becomes strong. Power has accumulated in this last folding in and, like a spring about to recoil, the foetus is ready to birth.

Birth itself, the passage through and out of the birth canal, will finally allow the infant to extend fully as they emerge out into the world.

7: Early Imprints

When the time is right, the foetus is called to initiate birth through releasing the hormone cortisol from its adrenal glands; this acts upon the placenta to increase oestrogen, which is registered by the mother's brain. Mother responds with a cascade of hormones that begin the labour. Whether they feel ready and willing or not, both must engage with the inevitability of birth.

Birth is one of the two greatest initiatory journeys that we will all be called to make in our lifetime. The other is the passage out of this embodied life at the time of death. In between are many transitions, rites of passage, crises, creative processes and inner and outer journeyings, each of which can mark a profound change from one way of being to another, one phase of life to the next. Our original birth experience lays down powerful imprints within cells, fluids and nervous system, which might be re-activated as we go through transitional and initiatory processes later in life. Becoming aware of how birth imprints might still be affecting our passage through life can be a powerful start to releasing limiting patterns, so that we can move forward with more freedom, whole-hearted courage, power and joy.

In my training programmes I developed a process of embodying the birth process where participants can re-experience the movements, sensations and feelings of birthing in a supported way. This is best done in a small group, though it is also possible to adapt the practice to work with individual clients in therapy when a birthing is called for (Hartley 2004: 124-5). During birth, mother and baby need layers of support around them – ideally partner, close family and friends, midwife, doctor, extended family and the wider community, the presence of Nature, maybe music and dance to support the rhythms of contraction and release. When re-embodying birth, working in a group can help to create this sense of layered support; a group also offers the experience of being witnessed in the momentous journey of birth by a 'family'. When the 'infant' emerges, they are greeted by mother and also by the wider community they have been born into.

Embodying the Birth Process

- ➤ Before re-creating the birth experience, students have been re-introduced to the movement patterns that offer underlying support and impetus for birthing:

    - they have embodied the *in-utero* patterns of *cellular breathing, navel radiation, pre-spinal* and *mouthing[1] patterns* of movement (see chapter 9: 145) (Hartley 1995; Bainbridge Cohen 2018; Stokes 2002)

    - explored the dynamics of *yield and push* and *reach and pull* as initiators of movement through the spine (see chapter 9: 149)

    - developed balanced muscle, organ and spinal cord tone through practising *physiological flexion and extension* (see chapter 10: 161)

    - and aligned womb (or womb-space for men), heart and brain as organic supports for integrated spinal movement, in readiness for a whole-hearted, fully embodied birth experience

    - they have also practised listening to their body and what it needs, to their feelings and what they are calling for, and have been introduced to a psychological map which can help them to orient and find meaning in their embodied experiences (described below).

- ➤ Each person who goes through the birth process is supported by a small group of about four or five people, who form a 'womb' around the birthing one. They have prepared by developing the capacity to hold a safe space for another with care, attentive listening, receptivity and compassion; they offer support and witnessing as they sit in a circle and enclose the birthing one. Gradually they come closer, making contact (with the birthing one's prior consent) and slowly increasing the pressure to simulate the narrowing of the space in the womb as the foetus grows. As the pressure intensifies, the birthing

> one will begin to respond, and together they can re-discover the rhythms of contraction and release

> The aims of re-embodying birth are two-fold: participants might learn about the personal meaning each stage and gesture of birthing holds for them, about the challenges, resources, feelings evoked, and patterns that were imprinted during their original birth; birth trauma might be re-activated and needs to be held with skill and care. Or they might experience something new, different from their original birth – a birth that is well-supported and full of shared power, love and joy perhaps. When someone has prepared well, worked through enough of their early trauma, become conscious of patterns imprinted in their cells and nervous system, they might now be ready to experience the full potential of a joyful and empowering birth within a sacred and well-held circle. It is possible to enter the process many times until there is readiness to experience this potential fully, imprinting a new pathway for future transitions that can offer more freedom and creative expression.

Grof's Basic Peri-Natal Matrix (BPM)

Radical psychiatrist Stanislav Grof experimented in the 1950s and 1960s with LSD, taking psychotic patients right into and through their process with the aim of releasing trauma locked into their psycho-physiological and spiritual system (Grof 1985, 1988). He documented a series of stages that he witnessed in thousands of accounts of these journeys; patients were re-enacting their birth experience through these consecutive stages and their descriptions can also be seen to mirror descriptions of the initiatory journeys of the shaman. The shaman dies to his old identity and is re-born into a new state of being; the birthing child dies to the old life in the womb and is born into a world of gravity, light and air, of clear sounds and new colours, smells and tastes, and relationship.

Grof was eventually arrested for the use of LSD in this work, but later developed methods to continue his research and therapy using techniques that include breath-work, massage and music[2]. Whilst I am not a practitioner of Grof's methods, I find his articulation of the stages of birth to be enlightening and very complementary to a somatic approach based on the Body-Mind Centering principles of infant movement development.

To further contextualise the birth experience, I integrate theory and practice from Psychosynthesis transpersonal psychotherapy[3], where I was first introduced to Stanislav Grof's model of the *Basic Peri-Natal Matrix* (BPM). This three-layered approach allows us to both orient within the often-powerful feelings evoked by re-embodying birth, and also to contextualise them in terms of personality development, our continuing experience as adults, and our unique way of engaging with Spirit as our life unfolds.

At each stage there is the potential for a self-affirming and life-affirming experience. There is also the potential for distress, trauma and difficulty in integrating the challenge of each stage. We will inevitably have a combination of good and bad experiences, but if the bad is not too extreme, prolonged or frequent, then a 'good enough' womb and birth can become imprinted within our cells and nervous system. This will lay a good foundation for healthy growth and development after birth and throughout life.

Each stage of the birth process embodies a specific quality, an aspect of our essential nature that holds both psychological and spiritual potentials. Negative experiences at each stage can lead to the distortion of these core qualities, and from these distortions *sub-personalities* develop as we grow towards adulthood (Ferrucci 1982: 47). Sub-personalities are semi-autonomous parts of the personality that can take over and feel as if they are the whole of who we are, rather than a part, a distortion of a quality and energy at the core of our being. This core energy is essentially good and healthy but has been blocked from expressing as it needs to. Spiritual qualities of harmony and peace, love and power are evoked through the stages of birth; when they cannot be experienced and expressed in a full and positive way, sub-personalities that can be named as the 'false mystic', 'victim' and 'rebel' might constellate. Identifying with one of these parts inhibits our connection with the whole of who we are, and limits the full expression of our true nature.

Later I will say more about being with challenging situations where disruption and trauma have caused splitting and more severe disturbances; for now, I will describe the main stages of actual birth and the ways they might be experienced when returned to as an adult and consciously embodied.

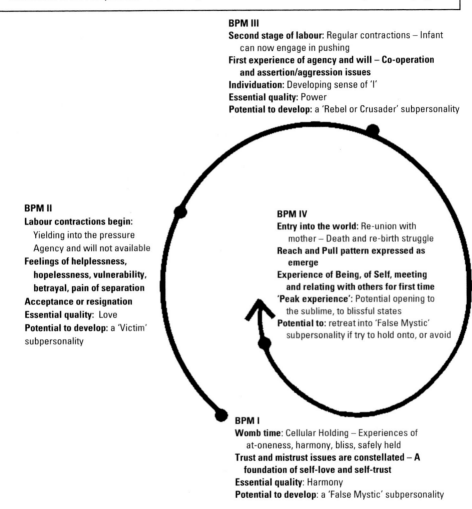

Figure 7.1: Spirallic Diagram of the Basic Perinatal Matrix

Womb Time, Eternal Time – BPM 1

The time spent in the womb, nestled away, both in the world and invisible to it, has been described by Frank Lake as "the womb of spirit" (Lake 1979). The relationship of Spirit with individual being, with other and with the world is gestating, finding a pathway to express, just as the embryonic, foetal and infant body is evolving and coming into form. Psychological and spiritual imprints are being laid down. Franklyn Sills writes:

> [During] the period from conception through the first nine months after birth ... the little one lives in womb-time, experiences his needs as though they are also mother's needs, and begins the shift from what Lake called being-in-relationship, the experience of being as mediated by mother's presence, to being-in-itself, a coherent and continuous experience of being not dependent on mother's reflection. (Sills 2009: 114)

If the womb feels 'good enough', experienced on the whole as positive, the foetus can yield into the holding, the constant nourishment and protection that is there. The womb is her whole world and she exists at the centre of this world. Sensations and feelings of peace, harmony and omnipotence become imprinted in the very cells and tissues. There is nowhere to go, nothing to be done or achieved – it is a time of Being rather than Doing. A state of blissful receptivity to the benevolence of the universe can lay the foundation for experiences of self-love and trust in a caring world to unfold, and this can serve as a strong root for the later unfolding of a spiritual life.

For some, the womb-time might be felt as blissful and some part of us wants to stay there, even as we progress through adult life. Some statements that might arise when we want to hold onto this stage are: 'everything is fine just as it is', 'I have everything I need, I don't need to engage, or change', 'let's not argue, I just want peace and harmony'.

The over-riding experience of the womb might be full of threat and toxicity though. An embryo and foetus is very sensitive and exposed to the unprocessed emotions of the mother and, through her, of the father and the wider society they live within. A mother who is stressed, anxious or depressed produces stress hormones which affect the foetus. Smoking, drugs and poor nutrition are also known to have detrimental effects. So too can the attitudes of the parents – if the mother or father does not want the child, for example, this message can be perceived by the foetus, creating an emotionally toxic womb environment. A message that the child is very much wanted can also be challenging to the foetus, and later the child, if great expectations are placed upon her even before birth. I have also worked with clients who have been conceived by a mother who is still grieving a previous lost child; this can have a deep and lasting impact on the child, who might have no idea where her own feelings of grief, anxiety or depression stem from. Feeling her own physical boundaries, her embodied form and her own breath become vital in the process of recovering her true self from enmeshment in the mother's grief. Feeling held within the therapeutic relationship, either literally through physical touch and holding, or emotionally through the compassionate witnessing presence of the therapist, the client may begin to experience a path towards freedom from all that has been absorbed from mother during gestation.

One way in which we might get caught at this stage is if it has felt not fulfilling enough, so we want more; or perhaps it has felt so perfect that we do not want to lose the experience of being safely and lovingly held in the womb as labour begins. We are not ready for the next stage when it arrives, and may resist the calling to be birthed. Or a toxic womb experience might lead us to want to get out just as soon as we can, to escape, to flee. All of these experiences, and more, can imprint patterns within us upon which personality development will evolve.

There are many ways in which the womb experience might not have given the foetus what she needs in order to embrace what comes next – the first stage of labour. The sacred qualities of peace, harmony, and the capacity to yield into pure Being are compromised and a 'false mystic' sub-personality might develop – this is the part of us that does not want conflict or challenge, that wants to stay in our 'meditation hut or cave', on our meditation cushion or yoga mat, not facing the gritty challenges of life and relationship, in order to maintain a rarefied sense of being-at-one with the Universe. Whilst a laudable aspiration for the genuine mystic who is ready for the gruelling path of spiritual awakening, the one who has not yet embraced the challenges of living may be thwarted in her attempts to stay above the fray and live in such an exalted state. Many western false mystics have been born since the arrival of spiritual practices from the East during the 1960s and beyond. Eventually we all need to come back down to the ground and learn to embody ourselves, as we come to terms with life as conscious beings of both matter and Spirit.

Whatever our experience of the "womb of spirit" was, we can all benefit from time spent returning to a place of safe and comfortable holding for a while. In a group or therapeutic setting, the practice of cellular touch (Hartley 1995: Ch 1) can be used to support an experience of deep relaxation, rest and return to self, simulating the cellular holding that is associated with the time in the womb. You can also try this on your own when you feel the need to rest or get away from it all, or as a daily practice of taking time out for yourself:

Nesting

- ➢ Carve out some time for yourself and retreat to a place that is comfortable, warm and undisturbed – this might be your bed, sofa, a mattress in the corner of the room. Have a bundle of blankets and cushions to hand. Curl up in the most comfortable way you can, using the cushions and blankets to make yourself as cosy and snug as possible.

- ➢ You might like to play some gentle and relaxing or inspiring music in the background. This can help to soften mental activity, allowing you to be more present to the moment.

- ➢ Rest and relax. Whenever you need to, adjust your position, move when you need to or rest in stillness.

- ➢ To help stop your thoughts from distracting you too much, bring your attention to the sensations of your breathing, your body weight yielding into the supporting surfaces, or the sounds you can hear. If you are familiar with the practice of cellular breathing, you can allow your attention to deepen into this.

- ➢ Rest, relax, soften, breathe, yield into the support beneath and surrounding you. And that is all, until you feel refreshed and ready to return to your day, or until you fall asleep.

I used to reflect often on my grandmother's life, on how, even before I was born, she had lived through two world wars, a pandemic and the Great Depression of the 1930s. My life in comparison had been relatively easy – not without challenge, stress and difficulties but on the whole, here in my home country of England, I was mostly held safe and secure from major collective disruption and trauma. In comparison to my grandmother's life and the lives of so many people in other parts of the world, I had lived in a safe place. Since the pandemic of 2020, and now the wars that are erupting ever closer to home, I realise that we had been gifted with a life of 'innocence' reminiscent of the womb space of BPM 1. This is not to negate or belittle the very real difficulties that we all experience, some more so than others, as we go through our lives; but collectively my generation, born post-war in the West, has been blessed with relative peace.

Paradise Lost – BPM 2

As the foetus grows to fill the whole space of the womb, he is compressed into a tightly curled foetal position. The pressure increases muscle, organ and spinal cord tone, readying the little one to play an active part in his birth. As labour begins, the walls of the womb begin to contract. In the first stage of labour the rhythm reflects the rhythm and motions of the digestive tract – sequential wave-like contractions through the powerful muscles of the womb that resemble the squeezing and releasing of digestive peristalsis. This wave-like rhythm can be witnessed in the person re-embodying birth, as the whole body begins to organise and orient towards engaging more fully with the direction of passage along the birth canal. The supporters of the re-birthing process offer resistance through their contact to whichever parts of the body are straining out beyond the firmly held boundary they are offering.

In searching for an image that might reflect this stage, my mind goes to what I imagine could be the experience of someone caught up in a large crowd surging towards a narrow or closed exit – a mass exodus of refugees, for example, fleeing a pressurised situation of war or conflict. Fear, chaos and confusion abound, with no sense of a safe escape route – a truly traumatising life-or-death situation. The more prosaic image of being swirled around in an overloaded washing machine might be another. Imagine, but please don't try this!

For the birthing infant there is not yet a clear sense of form and direction to these movements, no sense of the way out; rather, the experience can be of intolerable pressure bearing down from all directions. As the womb contracts, he needs to yield into this, then open, expand, adjust as the contraction releases; each contraction is building energy and power, and supports the organisation of the whole body for integrated movement in the next stage. A core of inner strength along the length of the spine, supported by the soft spinal cord at the back and digestive tract at the front, is being activated, so that he can engage and participate in his birth with agency. But how hard this can be, to yield into the pressure when it feels as if the whole world is crushing in on you and there is no way out, no escape or release. To resist, fight back, or collapse under the overwhelming pressure are all understandable responses.

How often in life do we feel like this? Some statements from this stage might be: 'everyone is against me', 'I'm stuck and there's no way out', 'there's no light at the end of the tunnel', 'everything is going wrong and there's nothing I can do about it', 'I feel helpless, hopeless'. If we have been unable to integrate the challenges of this stage of birth, and certainly this will be hard for many of us, feelings of being stuck and obstructed can remain central to our life experience, and identification as a victim may be the result.

In re-embodying the birth process in a group setting, the quality of support that is offered can help to free this sense of stuckness. Connection that is sensitive and responsive – to the subtlest of movements of the birthing one, to changes in their breathing, sounds, sighs, emotions expressed – is called for. With caring and attentive listening, a pathway can be found.

The challenge is to yield into the pressure and the rhythm of contraction and release, accepting that the contracting womb is an expression of a greater power, a greater love, that is impelling us to evolve, to make this momentous transition into a wholly new experience of life. Yielding into it means accepting, being with the pain and suffering. When we cannot do this, we may come to harbour resentment, hurt, feelings of betrayal, helplessness and, beneath this, anger. A 'victim' subpersonality is constellated.

This can be a very hard place to stay with. There is great uncertainty, not knowing if there really is a way out, or in which direction it might lie. I am writing this during the lockdown necessitated by the spread of the coronavirus. We are in a place of collective initiation, a potential re-birth of humanity into a new way of being on our planet Earth (or perhaps even elsewhere?) (Hartley 2020). How we move through this crisis may determine the sustainability and fairness of our future world. If we resist the restrictions that are being put on us now, like the birthing infant who cannot surrender to the constrictions of the first stage of labour, we may not be able to access the powerful and life-affirming potential of the second stage of labour, when the infant begins to push and find his own power and agency. Of course, mother as well as infant needs to be in a state of readiness and willingness; in our global situation, we need empathic and responsive leadership as well as empowered creative action from the people.

As with every birth process, our current collective crisis might or might not lead to the hoped-for new life. There is no guarantee of this and, around the world, corruption, greed and unresponsive leadership abound. Returning to this theme some time after I first drafted this section – after two appalling new wars have begun, further degradation of Nature, failures to prevent the climate crisis dangerously escalating, and injustice everywhere – hope hangs in the balance, held tentatively by some who continue to work hard towards the future they want to see, lost by others. Birth is indeed a life and death struggle.

Discovering Agency – BPM 3

We are not there yet in this collective transformation, the *Great Turning* as this time of collective and global change has been named by Joanna Macy (Macy & Johnstone 2012). Macy's work offers pathways to support us towards more resilience as we move through multiple crises of planetary, social and political upheaval. As we approach a new phase in our collective existence, perhaps in months or years, or maybe even decades ahead, we will face the question: can we work with what is, join with the greater forces acting upon us to create something new and beautiful? Or will the majority of us be rebelling against these forces, fighting one another, demanding individual rights when we need to focus on the wellbeing of the whole collective of humanity, Earth and Nature?

In the third stage of the basic peri-natal matrix we see the emerging of form as the *spinal patterns* integrate to initiate powerful whole-body movements between the head and tail of the spine. The contractions intensify and become more regular; they now follow the craniosacral rhythm as long, slow and deep muscle contractions through the length of the womb help to push the birthing infant down, towards the opening. She is called to alternate yielding into the contractions, with pushing through the birth canal as the contractions release. Now there is a sense of going somewhere, a light at the end of the tunnel towards which she can move. Agency, purpose and assertive, embodied power are the potentials of the second stage of labour.

If she has been able to release the potentially blissful paradise of the first phase, held securely in womb time, then accept and yield into the pressures and constrictions as labour begins, gathering a core of inner strength to propel her onwards, the birthing infant can now begin to engage actively in pushing her way through the birth canal. The potential of the second stage of labour is to work together with the contracting womb, to find shared rhythm and purpose as infant and mother yield and push in synchrony to birth the child.

When this can happen, the experience can be joyful, empowering and, for some, orgasmic. For many reasons this does not always, or even often, happen. The mother brings her own history of unresolved trauma, emotions, fears and expectations to the birth. There might be unnecessary intervention or lack of support from outside. And the child, too, brings that which is innate – her genetic tendencies and her 'karma'; in Buddhist psychology the term karma includes a predisposition to experience and respond to situations in particular ways, which we can carry with us from one lifetime to the next. Birth is the first time the infant meets the will of the *other* in a significant way, and innate tendencies and patterns, including those imprinted during conception and development *in utero*, can be activated. So rather than thinking of the birth experience as purely causal, we can see it as the first meeting of two beings, each with their own will and predispositions; they might join together in co-operation and mutual support or they might come into conflict. The birthing infant needs a mother who is ready to release her, then receive and welcome her anew.

When re-embodying birth within the supportive circle of a group, the pattern and rhythm of strong contraction and release through the length of the spine is clearly felt and witnessed. The womb-supporters must work hard to hold the container well enough for the birthing one to deeply experience the power of their movement and their agency. The integration of their core, from birthing crown of the head to tail of the spine and feet, becomes clear. The helpers increase the support and resistance at key points to maintain the womb-container, folding the birthing one back into the flexed position after each push, until the head finally and decisively breaks through.

Here is a simple way to experience the power of this movement on your own:

A movement practice to prepare for birthing

- ➤ Lie on your side on the floor – a non-resistant surface like wood is best for this – with your feet against the wall and your body flexed in as tightly as is comfortable.

- ➤ Taking the time you need to breathe into the movement, begin to push against the wall with your feet and allow the impulse to travel all the way up your legs, through your tailbone and along your spine. You will begin to unfold, lengthen, extend until your head is reaching into the space ahead. Keep in contact with your feet against the wall and your tailbone – the impulse for the movement comes from here.

➤ When you are fully extended, you can curl up again and repeat as many times as you like. Once you feel the movement integrates through your whole length you might find the power to go more quickly, or you might enjoy a slower rhythm where you can track the movement through each part of your body as it extends. Let your breathing support you.

➤ Afterwards stand and simply notice how you feel – in particular, how do the contact of the soles of your feet with the floor and your vertical alignment around your centre feel?

In a positive passage through this stage, the infant can experience self-assertion and power as something life-affirming and life-enhancing. The capacity to act in co-operation with the greater forces of life that are birthing the infant gives her power rather than taking it away. She knows that she has agency and will, and when she can align her will with that of others, and ultimately with that which we might call Universal will – a divine force that flows through each of us – then her power can be effective and creative. Returning to our embodied self enables us to re-connect to this relationship between personal and Universal will, and to know more clearly how to *yield into*, so that choices and directions in life become clear.

So many factors contribute to the experience of the third stage of the matrix, as we have explored. When the infant and mother are not able to come into a reciprocal relationship of shared rhythm, support and intention, the birthing infant might feel the impulse to panic or fight against, instead of move with the contracting womb. The potential for power to be distorted into anger, aggression and unwillingness, or inability, to co-operate can lead to the development of a 'rebel' sub-personality, an 'outsider' or a 'crusader' who goes through life believing that their way is the right and only way, and will impose it on others no matter the cost. An unintegrated BPM 3 can lead to all manner of oppressive, abusive and conflictual relationships in the world, as we can see everywhere around us.

The Threshold between Life and Death, Joy and Existential Anxiety – BPM 4

The last stage marks the emergence from the birth canal. After hours of yielding into and pushing through, the head (or the body part that is leading the way, sometimes the pelvis or legs, or a shoulder) breaks through the constraints of the birth canal with a mighty *reach and pull* impulse as it is freed. The infant is born into a completely new world of air and Earth and other. The promise of the fourth stage of the peri-natal matrix is of a joyful re-union between mother and little one, when the pain of the birth has been met, yielded into, accepted and worked through, mother and infant in synchronised rhythms of contraction and release. It can be experienced as a profoundly spiritual as well as emotional moment for both. The risk is that, instead, the infant feels the total loss of his known world in the womb as death and annihilation; anxiety, traumatic stress and conflict can result.

This stage is not thought to engender a sub-personality constellation, but will have deep implications for development through infancy, childhood and into adulthood. If experienced as a moment of joyful union, the little one is gifted with the laying down of an imprint of loving relationship that can support him throughout his life. But perhaps he will grow into an adult who wants to hold onto the 'high' and live forever in blissful harmony. Like the game 'snakes and ladders', he is then right back at the beginning of the cycle as a 'false mystic' sub-personality is constellated.

A negative birth experience can have an even wider and far-reaching impact on the individual's future development. Birth is undoubtedly stressful for the infant, and it is intended to be: during periods of moderate stress, enormous levels of learning and neurological development are taking place; and the intense friction of skin against the walls of the birth canal during the hours of labour have the effect of stimulating vital organ systems such as the digestive, immune, endocrine and respiratory systems. Other mammals fulfil this function by licking their infant after birth; the effect is the same – the stimulation of essential physiological processes that prepare the infant for life in his new environment outside the womb (Montagu 1986). He must now learn to breathe air into and out of his lungs, digest his own food, develop an immune system capable of protecting him from many kinds of assaults, and gradually evolve the capacity to regulate his own responses to inner and outer changes and demands. Birth is just the beginning, but it lays down imprints for how these processes, and many more, will develop through a lifetime.

Stress comes to play a detrimental part when it is too extreme, excessive, long-lasting and is not mitigated and resolved after the birth. In the post-partum phase both infant and mother need time to rest and recover in intimate connection, ideally skin to skin; loving relatedness supports oxytocin to be released, which aids the restoration of a sense of wellbeing for both. Breast-feeding also releases oxytocin, the 'love hormone'[4]. The autonomic nervous system, which has been profoundly activated by the birth stress, needs to re-balance so that the infant can integrate healthy cycles of activity and rest. When this does not happen well enough, post-traumatic stress pathways become imprinted in the brain and nervous system, in the cells and tissues of the body, and many physiological and psychological symptoms can evolve from this.

Reflections

Later we will look at some of the ways that somatic movement practice can support the re-balancing of the nervous system following unresolved birth (or other kinds of) stress. To end, I invite you to reflect on what you might know, or not know, about the stages of your own birth process and how it might still be playing out in your life as your system seeks healing and balance. In particular, you might find the imprints of birth patterning being re-activated during life transitions – periods of change, loss, learning or creative processes, for example.

These questions are simply guidelines to help you to reflect on the imprint of your birth and how it might still be impacting your life in the present. Add your own questions, change them, respond only to what feels useful and significant for you, and take time – you can simply hold a question that calls to you and see what arises over time. Or take your question into movement and see what your body wants to say about it; insight might arise. Go gently – take one part at a time. It would be helpful to share your reflections with someone else if you can. If strong emotions come up that you cannot comfortably hold or safely express, pause the exploration and consider seeking professional support to help you process and integrate what is arising. This might particularly be the case if your birth involved medical intervention, such as Caesarean section or forceps; exploring within a safe therapeutic relationship could be very beneficial.

Reflection on your birth process

Part 1

- You might have experience of some form of rebirthing work; but if you do not, you probably hold some ideas about your birth. Perhaps you have been told things by your mother or other family members; maybe you have fantasies about how it was for you. All of this can be useful information.

- Write down what you know, feel and imagine about your birth. Include anything you know or feel about your mother's experience of the birth, how other family members responded and any messages you feel you received from that time.

- Did you have to make a 'promise' or 'contract' with your mother in order to be born? (For example, 'I will be good, quiet, entertaining, helpful … if you will keep me, love me, cherish me.') Or perhaps you rebelled against any pressures or injunctions you felt were there. (Such promises might have emerged in embryonic form during conception or the time in the womb, and might be reinforced at birth and during various stages of childhood.)

Part 2

- Make yourself comfortable and take a few moments to follow the movements of your breathing, to settle and centre your mind within your body. With each breath the invitation is to deepen towards a still place of awareness within, so that the mind can soften and feelings and insights from deeper layers can arise.

- Imagine that your life is set out before you, like a film. Begin to watch as the story unfolds, being aware of important times of transition, learning, creative projects, life changes etc. Try not to get involved in the emotions – simply witness the unfolding story. And do not get caught up in the details – simply notice the pattern of events, then move on.

- You can also draw this as a timeline, marking the significant moments of your life from conception and birth to the present[5].

- Are you aware of a pattern in the way you dealt with these significant events and how the world responded to you?
- Within this pattern, do you see a place where you had difficulty, felt stuck, disempowered, lost or in some way frustrated or distressed?
- Do you see a place where you felt good, empowered, supported?
- Can you recognise any issues you have in relation to:
    1. the development and expression of your will – including the development of trust, the acceptance of limitations, your power to act and your willingness to be present and visible? Is there some place where your will may be unsupported, inhibited, weak, distorted or undeveloped?
    2. your patterns of change, learning or creativity throughout your life and in the present?
- Write some notes to anchor what came up for you.

Part 3

- Breathe and settle again.
- Where are you now in your life, in relation to cycles of change or growth – are you in a process in your life where something new is emerging, or perhaps something is completing and ending? How is it this time? Are you moving ahead, feeling stuck, lost, empowered, unclear?
- At which stage do you feel yourself to be in this cycle now:
    1. in a place where you are held and not too much is being demanded of you; perhaps there is a feeling of not-knowing or disconnection here
    2. in a situation where you feel under pressure, stuck, limited or constricted by circumstances that feel beyond your control; whatever you try to do, you feel unable to change your situation
    3. actively working through issues – engaged, pushing, asserting, battling, creating – to find a way through or complete something

4. released into a new place, a new way of being and being seen or of perceiving life, a new attitude, renewed energy, a project completed.

➢ What do you feel about what you are experiencing? How effective is your will in this situation? Do you feel supported or do you need something from outside? Do you have the resources within you to be fully present to this moment in your life? Are there any other questions you want to ask?

➢ Write some notes to anchor what came up for you.

➢ Drawing, dancing or other creative expressions can be very helpful in integrating or further exploring your experience.

8: Meeting the World

Buddhist psychology proposes that before birth we have consciousness of who we are and where we have come from, but that the intensity of the birth experience causes us to forget. From my explorations into re-embodying pre- and peri-natal processes, and those of students and clients I have worked with, I feel the truth of this. A quality of awareness and knowing seems to be present *in utero* and can be remembered during embodied explorations of pre-natal life. We can sense a glimmer, a trace of this in the newborn too – doting grandparents might be heard to say, "Ah, she's an old soul, she's been here before", as they recognise a quality that feels like a deep and ancient knowing. It is easy to feel that the newborn has an innate connection to Spirit, to the place she has come from, beyond the material world she must now learn to live within.

This sense of knowing seems in stark contrast to the consciousness of the totally dependent little one who has emerged into the world, who must now gradually learn to master her interactions with all she is about to encounter. There are so many things to learn, challenges to meet, skills to be mastered. No wonder we forget where we have come from and the knowing that we bring from that realm, as we are confronted with all the requirements of growing. No wonder we can lose direct connection to Spirit as the necessity of relating to our particular corner of life requires us to develop psychological structures that will enable us to become functioning adults in a material and social world.

Ashley Montagu proposes that a human infant is born half way through gestation (Montagu 1986: 53-4). If we compare our own development with that of other mammals, we see young pups, kittens, foals and cubs able to stand up, totter to the nipple and feed unaided within minutes of birth. It will take a human infant about nine months to reach the same degree of development and mastery, when she will finally be able to crawl to reach the object of her desire and need or retreat from what threatens her. One notable exception to this is a newborn who is allowed to crawl up her mother's belly and find the nipple immediately after birth, but this is a primitive instinctive action. She has not yet truly mastered the skill of crawling and will need help to meet her own needs for many months and years to come.

This acute dependency is balanced, however, by the marvellous plasticity of the human brain. Because so many basic functions still need to be learned after birth, within the rich and varied environment of the world of family and community, Earth, gravity and air, there are many opportunities for individual paths of development and creative adaptations. This has both advantages and disadvantages: there is greater potential for complex and creative learning and development, but also more possibilities for things to go wrong. We have greater freedom, choice and therefore also *response-ability* as human beings.

The infant has already 'met' the realities of her mother and father figure while in the womb; the pattern of her relationships with them began to form there, as we have explored, and it is likely that they will continue in a similar vein as she comes to know her parents in the new milieu of social interaction. The roots of attachment styles and imprints already laid down before and during birth are often reinforced. So powerful are these early imprints that they will colour our experience of what comes next, whatever the world offers us or confronts us with. If we have constellated a false mystic, victim or rebel approach to life we will meet whatever greets us after birth through this lens.

Grof describes the emergence of COEX systems, where *patterns of experiencing* are repeated throughout many stages of life until awareness of the pattern can be made conscious, and healing and resolution found (Grof 1985: 97). For the infant, sensitive, loving and therapeutic interventions can go a long way towards mitigating a negative pre- and peri-natal experience. On the other hand, adverse life circumstances can layer over what has been an essentially good beginning, compromising the infant and child's development. But positive earliest imprints can still be re-discovered as resources and supports for healing.

Sometimes a client in therapy must search a long way back to find the resources, the places of loving support and safety, that are needed to initiate a healing journey. A client or student exploring embryonic and foetal stages of development might find that there were experiences very early on, before later disruption and trauma, which can serve as potent resources. Re-embodying early places that are discovered to be supportive and integrating can help us to centre, ground, heal ruptured boundaries and return to presence when faced with later challenging or overwhelming events.

Embodiment of nurturing stages within the embryological journey, some of them described in previous chapters, can offer deep nourishment and holding, allowing distress and trauma to be met with safety. (More will be said about this in the following chapters.) Sometimes this means going right back to when we were no more than an energetic vibration, a potential, not yet embodied in matter; the roots of our spiritual longing can be felt to connect back to this source.

Emergence and Separation from the Ground of Being

The rupture of birth, whether empowering or deeply traumatic for the newborn, separates him from the state of oceanic bliss experienced in the womb, but not completely. For the first two months of post-natal life, he will spend much of his time in states of absorption, immersed in the *Dynamic Ground,* as it has been named by Michael Washburn (2003) – the foundation of psychic life where the newborn's consciousness is experienced as at-one with his universe. This primordial ground lies beneath and beyond the control of the ego; it is the plenipotent source of "energies, instinctual impulses, emotive currents, and images" (Washburn 2003: 38) that manifest within the psyche but are rooted in the physicality of soma, thus bridging psyche and soma. Washburn's description of the Dynamic Ground seems congruent with Jung's *collective unconscious*, the powerful source of experience that is common to the whole of the human species. Towards the end of his career Jung came to recognise that archetypes, which arise from the collective unconscious, have their roots within soma; they have organic, visceral, instinctual origins (Conger 1988: 185). Washburn writes:

> *At the outset of life we are radically open and, consequentially, receptive not only to a wide range of external stimuli but also to a wide range of energies, impulses, feelings, and images arising from the Dynamic Ground within.* (2003: 41)

It is my sense that the Dynamic Ground described by Washburn is resonant with what I have named elsewhere as the *ground of being* (Hartley 2001: 137). When in contact with this 'ground', which lies beneath the expressions of personality and self, we are in direct contact with Spirit. In a similar vein Franklyn Sills describes a three-layered mapping, informed by a Buddhist perspective, of *Source, Being, Self:*

> *Source – A numinous ground of emptiness from which Being arises and is ever connected*
>
> *Being – A locus, or coalescence, of awareness and meaning, the still centre in the midst of self-conditions*
>
> *Self – The substrate through which Being manifests, Self is both conditioned and conditioning* (Sills 2009: 7)

Seeing the Source or Dynamic Ground as a "numinous ground of emptiness", from which all manifestations of Being and Self arise, enables us to map human experience of the personal arising out of the universal, personal self as an expression of, or differentiation out of, universal Spirit. In this view, rooted in Buddhist and other mystical practices, Source or Spirit is boundless, empty of form, and also the potent ground out of which all form is endlessly arising. I make these theoretical comparisons not to lay down a definitive naming of the invisible worlds within and around us, but simply to orient and offer a loose approximation of the territory. I encourage the reader to follow their own instinct and insight when finding maps and names for the invisible and ineffable realms of experience.

With birth, the universe expands beyond the confines of the womb-world, but the infant has not yet separated himself from the Dynamic Ground and continues to experience self and world as one. The potential for merging with, or absorption within, the universal ground of consciousness remains with each of us throughout life, though it may only express in particular moments and situations, and most often not as the fully immersed and surrendered experience of the foetus and newborn. For the newborn and infant, the maternal figure is experienced as at-one with the Dynamic Ground, the source of all potentials within himself. As the Great Mother she embodies the immense power of this Ground, which has both a positive aspect – the Good Mother, nurturing and bountiful; and a terrifyingly threatening aspect – the Bad Mother (Washburn 2003: 43). (We can see how misogyny might later develop in someone who has not been able to integrate this negative power within himself.)

In this radically open state, there is as yet no clear experience of boundary separating the newborn from the world he now inhabits, and in particular from the maternal figure. He must begin to differentiate a *sense of self* in order to develop the ego functions that will enable him to master the series of challenges that lead towards independent living. To do this he will need to repress the potency of the Dynamic Ground and separate himself from the overwhelming power of the Great Mother. This is essential, at least for an infant born into a modern western culture; but it also necessitates a gradual loss or weakening of the experience of interconnectedness with the Universal, the *web of life* and the potency of the Dynamic Ground as Source of life. Over the coming years he will gradually come to know himself as a separate individual with a body, desires, needs, emotions and opinions that he identifies with as *self*. Everything and everyone else will be experienced as *other*. Certain aspects of himself that are rejected as too threatening or unacceptable will also come to be felt as *other*, as the *shadow* (Jung) or *disavowed self* (Stern). And so, his original sense of being-at-one with the Universe, wholly embedded in the ground of being and touched by Spirit, must be abandoned in favour of greater independence and individuation.

This is not necessarily the case within indigenous tribal cultures who live close to the Earth and Nature, where each infant is embedded within the web of community and a sense of place in ways that we have lost in modern society. Rooted in, supported and nourished by the whole community, the membrane that separates self from other remains permeable so that each individual continues to experience himself intimately connected to and a living part of the *web of life* – the whole of the natural world as well as his own tribe or village community. We will return to this theme later.

Whether tightly boundaried or fluidly open and receptive to the world beyond, a sense of self, as Stern has shown, develops out of the infant's sensory-motor processes and the affects which are layered within them (Stern 1985). Although Stern does not name the pre-natal experience as a foundation for the developing sense of self, the sensory-motor feedback loops that are the foundation for neurological growth have already begun to evolve *in utero*; hence we can infer that a sense of self is already *emerging* before birth.

From the perspective of Body-Mind Centering practice we can go back even further to say that a *pre-conscious sense of self* begins with the experience we name *cellular awareness*. From the very beginning, the fertilised cell is thought to have pre-conscious awareness of itself, as does every differentiated cell of the growing body; this can be experienced through the process of *visualisation, somatisation and embodiment,* as outlined earlier. This is a foundation of Body-Mind Centering embodied awareness practice. For a fully conscious sense of self to develop, the growth and maturation of the nervous system and brain, through sensory-motor processing, will be needed.

Francis Mott (1959) claims that the constant touch of amniotic fluids that swirl around the foetus sends a stream of sensory information from the membrane of the skin to the centre of the brain, the *hypothalamus*, and this flow of sensory stimulus creates the sense of being a centre with a periphery. A sense of core self and body boundary begin to constellate *in utero*; though the sense of self is merged with the universe of womb/mother and boundaries are highly permeable, the foetus experiences himself as the centre of this universe. The rhythmical surge of blood through the umbilical cord out from and into the foetal body also generates embryonic feelings such as aggressive penetration and empowerment, alternating with feeling victim to penetration, hollowed out and occupied, claims Mott from his study of clients' dreams (1959: 21).

From her observation of the movement interactions of pairs of twins in the womb and for several years after birth, Alessandra Piontelli has also shown that the development of a sense of self is already underway *in utero* (1992). Through her fascinating study, each twin is seen to express a unique personality *in utero*, which continues uninterrupted during and after birth. In one set of twins, it is observed that one of the pair dominates, with much kicking and elbowing of the other who tends to be less assertive. Another pair show tenderness, with one often caressing the other through the veil of their amniotic sacs. Such patterns of interaction were seen to continue immediately after birth and during the next five years of the study.

The subjective experience of being a *self*, a unique individual existing at the centre of a (largely) benevolent universe, which that self can surrender to and dissolve into or differentiate out of, is at the root and heart of the experience of being human. It is also at the heart of spiritual experience, which the individual might access at a later turn of the spiral as consciousness evolves. Connection to the Dynamic Ground, which has roots in soma, is the source of such later experiences of embodied spirituality, claims Washburn. The health, permeability, receptivity, rigidity or rupturing of the psychological membrane that embraces the self may greatly influence the way that Spirit is encountered. And, as we saw earlier, the intimate connection between the membranes that form the womb-container – two from the embryo's own tissue and the outer layer from the mother – must surely have bearing upon the relationship between self, other and ultimately Spirit.

Relational Consciousness

Human beings are relational – we are social creatures in need of relationship not only to thrive, but to survive. As interdependent beings, we are deeply connected to the whole of life and most immediately with other human beings whom we are closest to. The infant's brain, and with it her emerging sense of self, develops through relatedness with others. In the 1980s harrowing accounts of abandoned children, left without caring relationship and physical touch in Romanian orphanages, alerted the world to the profound damage, both physical and psychological, caused by lack of human connection. In his seminal book *Touching – The Human Significance of the Skin* (1971, 1986), Ashley Montagu records many instances of touch deprivation and its consequences for children and young animals. An infant and young child needs to be held, caressed, engaged with in face-to-face communication and play, offered steady eye contact and meaningful connection in order for her brain to develop as it is designed to.

The nervous system works through the passing of impulses over a space, the *synapse*, between two nerve cells; multiplied trillions of times, this action is a foundation of all neurological processing. In an analogous way, the relational space between humans has been called the *social synapse* (Cozolino 2006: 4); this relational space enables direct communication between an infant and her caregiver and is crucial to the infant's learning about self and other. Differentiating herself out of the primordial ground so that her individual selfhood can emerge is one of the first tasks of psychological growth and it happens within relationship to a caring other, or others, who are present, receptive and responsive to the infant's expressions and needs.

We saw earlier how the first polarity to emerge after conception, after the polar energies of *masculine and feminine* come together, is that of an *inner and outer* world. All that is contained within the membrane of the fertilised cell is associated with self and all that exists outside of it will come to be known as other. The cellular membrane is a highly sensitive and intelligent organ, determining what to allow into the cell as nourishment and energy, and what to release as waste or as chemical messengers that communicate with other cells.

In the months after birth the infant gradually learns to recognise a distinction between self and other, to know the centre of consciousness that is *I*, as differentiated from *Thou* and all that is *other*. In doing this, she both separates herself out from inherent connection with the *web of life* and at the same time brings herself into relationship to it in a new *dialogic* way – the perception of duality emerges. This necessary challenge allows her to develop and grow as an individual, but also gradually cuts her off from her previous direct connection with the Source of life, with Spirit and the Dynamic Ground from which her consciousness is differentiating.

This process is accelerated as language develops. As David Abram has shown, the evolution of abstract symbols to signify meanings replaced earlier forms of communication which were sensorily based, rooted in the embodied sense of being in relation to Nature and the geography of place. He writes:

> *If we listen, first, to the sounds of an oral language – to the rhythms, tones, and inflections that play through the speech of an oral culture – we will likely find that these elements are attuned, in multiple and subtle ways, to the contour and scale of the local landscape, to the depth of its valleys or the open stretch of its distances, to the visual rhythms of the local topography.* (140)
>
> *For ... numerous indigenous, oral cultures – the coherence of human language is inseparable from the coherence of the surrounding ecology, from the expressive vitality of the more-than-human terrain. It is the animate earth that speaks; human speech is but a part of that vaster discourse.* (Abram 1997, 2017: 179)

As the child born into a modern westernised culture learns to read and write using these abstract symbols, her innate sense of connection with Nature and Earth is inexorably diluted until she might come to feel entirely separate from the ground that is her home, and *other* in relation to the multitude of species we share our earthly home with. Sadly this often includes separation from her own animal nature, her embodied home.

The polarity of self and other, inner and outer, first delineated by the original cell membrane, is now embodied in the membrane of the skin. Like the cell membrane, the skin has two principal layers, one facing inwards and the other facing outwards. Information flows both ways – from the world outside to the innermost reaches of the central nervous system and brain, conveying information about the world; and from the brain out to the skin surface, changing the tone, colour, moistness or dryness, health and general appearance of the skin, expressing the internal conditions. Touch to the skin both nurtures the brain, helps it to grow, and also invites the inner self to open out to meet the world, to express itself in the world. Nurturing and appropriate touch is essential to the healthy development of the sense of self and its expression.

During the lockdowns necessitated by the pandemic we were told NOT to get too close to each other, as is our natural, healthy instinct in times of stress or hardship; not to touch or receive the touch that would normally sustain our health and wellbeing, and the fabric of family and social life. As a result of this enforced denial of an essential need, both physical and mental health have been sorely challenged for many people. We wait to see what the long-term consequences of this might be.

Besides nerve pathways, intricate webs of connection run throughout the body – fibres of *connective tissue* weave from the layers of the skin, around and within all the body tissues and organs, and right into the heart of each cell. Microscopic fibres pass into each cell and even its nucleus, creating an internal *cytoskeleton* which supports the structure and functioning of the cell (Oschman 2000: 43-50). This network carries information directly from the skin right into the heart of every single cell of the body; information is conveyed directly to the DNA which regulates the cell's activity, and thus the whole body's functioning. Our health is directly affected by the quality and amount of touch our skin receives.

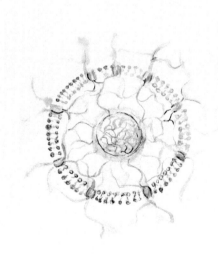

Figure 8.1: Two-layered cell membrane and cytoskeleton.
Artist: Raima Drąsutytė

The connection between inner and outer, mediated through the skin, joins our inner being in an intimate dance with the world outside. The skin as an interface between inner and outer is an organ of communication, transformation and connection. When in healthy balance it offers a clear, responsive and protective boundary, as well as a means of establishing intimate relationship with the world we live in. Out of the skin and nervous system the special senses (taste, smell, hearing and sight) also develop, enabling more specific and detailed ways of sensing the outer world. Proprioceptive and interoceptive nerves provide pathways to sense our inner world.

A healthy boundary contains an integrated sense of self which is also open and receptive to the world in which self is embedded; this interface is both the physical reality of the skin and the psychological awareness of the relationship between self and other. Maintaining the integrity and heath of this membrane of awareness is one of the challenges we all face throughout the whole of our lives.

Bodywork and massage are wonderful ways to receive nurturing through touch, strengthening the protective and integrative functions of the skin. When this is not available, we can nurture ourselves through the *touch of attention*; using mindful movement explorations to nourish our skin membrane, we can strengthen a healthy sense of clear and responsive boundary, an interface between inner and outer. You might like to try this exploration:

An Exploration – the meeting of skin with ground

- ➢ Find a comfortable place to lie down. A firm surface, with a soft covering if you need it, is ideal; outside, lying on grass or sand, can feel especially nourishing; or at home on your bed if that feels best, maybe in those times when illness limits other possibilities.

- ➢ Allow yourself a few moments to rest and relax, inviting your body to spread into the ground, yielding weight and feeling the movement of your breath.

- ➢ Take your attention to the surfaces of your body that are in contact with the ground and simply notice what you sense and feel there.

You can scan through your body, from head to feet or feet to head, noticing where you are able to yield your weight more fully into the Earth and where maybe the contact is less clear and there is some withholding of weight. Do not judge – simply witness, breathe and let go.

- ➤ When you feel an impulse to move, to shift, change your position, allow this to happen – it might begin with a simple rolling of your head or stretching of a limb. Follow movement that feels easy, allowing yourself to roll, stretch, slide, curl and uncurl.

- ➤ As you move, seek to keep your attention with the places where your skin is touching the ground, directly or through clothing. Follow the contact of skin with ground, inviting your skin to spread out to meet the surface and your weight to release through each new place of contact so that your connection to the Earth deepens with each shift.

- ➤ Rest whenever you wish to, softening into the Earth through the places of contact. Then begin moving again when you are ready, letting the meeting of skin and ground be a place of both support and initiation for the movement. Find your own rhythm between moving and resting.

Mediating Inner and Outer through the Autonomic Nervous System

In utero, the foetal brain has been developing in preparation for life beyond the womb. Birth initiates an immense surge in the growth and increasing complexity of the human brain. The stress of birth creates massive new connections between neurons, which enable great leaps of learning to take place; and the friction of passage through the birth canal stimulates organ systems such as the respiratory, digestive and immune systems in preparation for survival in the world the newly born has emerged into. Rapid development continues throughout the first few years of life. However, it will be some time before the *cortex* is functioning and has matured enough to enable consciousness to fully emerge. Before this can happen, the infant swims in a pre-conscious state of awareness, mediated primarily by low-brain and mid-brain centres.

Before conscious awareness and intentional control develop, physiological and psychological function is largely co-ordinated through the *autonomic nervous system* (ANS), interlaced with hormonal and chemical feedback loops that integrate the brain with all of the body systems. As the name describes, the autonomic nervous system works through non-intentional, autonomic processes which are, for the most part, beyond our control, though influenced by both conscious and unconscious thought and emotion. The infant is still dominated by the power and depth of the Dynamic Ground out of which he is gradually differentiating. Psychoanalysts describe a process of *primal repression*, which allows the infant and young child to manage the potentially overwhelming power of the ground of being as the ego develops and the infant begins to gain some measure of mastery over himself and his world (Washburn 2003: 44-6).

At a neurological level, primal repression is dependent on maturation of the *orbito-prefrontal cortex,* which enables modulation of the autonomic nervous system; through this, the infant gradually acquires the capacity to regulate impulses, drives, emotions and instinctual behaviours. Through this process, he represses the potentially overwhelming power of the Dynamic Ground, which becomes relegated to the shadows until developments later in life trigger its resurgence. For example, aspects of it can erupt during puberty and adolescence, during sexual orgasm, in giving birth, when traumatised, grieving deeply, during mental breakdown or when profoundly engaged in creative process; and, for some, during experiences of spiritual awakening or *spiritual emergency* (Grof & Grof 1989).

Like the original cell membrane, then the skin, the autonomic nervous system embodies the polarity of *inward and outward facing*, evolving as a complex and nuanced system to regulate the internal needs of the infant in relationship to external demands and changing conditions. It consists of two branches, the *parasympathetic* and *sympathetic*, which ideally work together in a complementary way, counterbalancing each other to maintain the health and wellbeing of both soma and psyche (Bainbridge Cohen 2008: 175; Hartley 2004: 163-5). A healthy and balanced nervous system alternates between the two in cyclical or wave-like rhythms.

There are also two parts to the parasympathetic branch: the oldest part, which is mediated by the *dorsal vagal nerve*, supports *inward-focused attention* and processes of rest, digestion, absorption and recuperation. It enervates organs below the diaphragm and primarily increases activity in those involved in digestion. With parasympathetic activation, alertness to the world outside is diminished; engagement with the inner workings of the body and psyche are heightened and states of peace and calm can be experienced. The newborn is very much engaged with processing in these ways and the *vegetative parasympathetic nervous system* is dominant in the earliest months of life. It is the ground for physiological functioning, as well as states of pure being and awareness. A foundation for embodied presence, it invites states of *beingness*, before the differentiations of specific *doings* begin to manifest.

The sympathetic nervous system faces outward. It evolved in vertebrates that needed to develop skills to actively negotiate threat and danger, hunt and develop more complex engagement with their environment. *Attention is focused outwards*, with the eyes and ears wide open to the outside world, muscles readied for action by neural activation and adrenalin; there is a heightened state of alertness and vigilance. In everyday life, we need some measure of sympathetic activation to get out of bed in the morning and prepare to meet the demands of our day. It supports us to meet challenges, achieve goals, interact creatively with our world, compete or extend ourselves in work, sport and other activities. If the sympathetic nervous system remains connected to and grounded in the vegetative parasympathetic nervous system, then activity is supported and we can easily and periodically return to restful states to regenerate when needed.

During the 1990s Stephen Porges' research brought to light another aspect of the parasympathetic nervous system. An evolutionary development of the *vagus nerve*, the tenth cranial nerve which activates the parasympathetic system, was discovered. Called the new *ventral vagal nerve*, it activates systems above the diaphragm, including the heart, breathing, expressive facial muscles, the vocal mechanism, eyes and hearing (Porges 2011). This nerve and the complex of functions it co-ordinates have been named the *social engagement system* (SES); activation of the social engagement system is a primary way in which mammals seek safety when the environment is experienced as threatening or dangerous; it has been called the *tend and befriend* response, in distinction from the *fight or flight* and *freeze* responses.

The social engagement system enables co-regulation between humans, and between other mammals, so that during dangerous or stressful situations hyperarousal (sympathetic nervous system activation) and hypoarousal (vegetative parasympathetic nervous system activation) can be calmed and feelings of safety and balance restored. During social interaction, direct face-to-face and eye contact, the tone of voice and expressiveness of the face all communicate over the social synapse in a language that is beyond words; it is not the meaning of the words so much as the quality of engagement, expressed through an integrated breath-heart-face-eyes-ears-voice system, which enables nervous system regulation to be restored. The ventral vagal nerve complex simultaneously activates all of these social functions. Through it we express and perceive empathy, compassion, kindness and other calming, reassuring communications that help to soothe and regulate the over-activated nervous system.

My brother-in-law recently sent me a video he had taken of his seven-month-old grandson as he played a game of 'looking, looking away'. As they connected, the little one immediately lit up, full of joy and excitement, laughing, 'singing', smiling and kicking in sheer delight. The moment his grandad looked away a faint shadow passed over the little one's eyes, he stopped laughing and dancing. He waited patiently, still and attentive, for connection to return; an expression that perhaps hinted at loss or confusion momentarily replaced the joy, until grandad returned his gaze and the little one immediately lit up again. It was such a striking example of the effect of social engagement on the infant's whole psychological and physiological being, and the contrasting impact of the lack of it. To experience fully embodied wellbeing, health of body and mind, and feelings of safety and security, the infant needs social engagement; through it, he grows his young brain and cultivates the capacity to form loving relationships throughout life. When deprived of this beyond his endurance it is easy to see how the hint of a shadow of loss and confusion could develop into significant emotional and psychological suffering later in life. Games of 'looking and looking away', or hide-and-seek, enable the little one to learn that loved ones may temporarily disappear, but will soon return.

Porges' work showed that there is a hierarchy of defensive processes which we reach for when safety is threatened. When available, a healthy response is to seek social engagement with those who can help us to regulate and feel safe again. If this is not available or appropriate, or if earlier trauma has imprinted unhealthy patterns of dysregulation within the autonomic nervous system, we might resort to the hyperarousal state of a *fight or flight* response. The fight or flight response to threat, challenge, stress or danger is mediated through the sympathetic branch of the autonomic nervous system. If this fails, or if habitual patterning has already determined this pathway, we descend into a state of hypoarousal that can lead to dissociation, numbness, collapse, despair or depression, a *freeze* response. This is as true for the young infant as for the child or adult.

As a primitive line of defence against threat, reptiles, amphibians and mammals, including humans, developed the freeze response, 'playing dead' in the face of extreme threat or danger; this response is mediated through the dorsal vagal complex, the vegetative parasympathetic nervous system. It might be resorted to when other processes have failed. Think of a toad being uncovered from its hiding place, turning to 'stone' to avoid detection; or a mouse 'playing dead' when caught by a cat in the hope the cat loses interest, only wanting to experience the chase and not the feast. When our nervous system is overwhelmed by threatening stimulus, we fear for our life or safety and cannot access another way of responding in the moment, we humans too might freeze, shutdown and withdraw into ourselves.

If we have learnt to be mindful in the moment that we begin to feel overwhelmed, we might be able to withdraw out of choice as we seek to resource ourselves through mindful breathing, body awareness, a walk by the sea or in the woods, or a few hours under the duvet, for example. But if we cannot emerge from it, periods of withdrawal can lead to psychological and physiological shutdown, dissociation, collapse into inertia and depression, and eventual ill-health might develop. This is in essence a protective response of the old parasympathetic nervous system, but can lead to pathologies when we are unable to fully return from it. In his seminal book *Waking the Tiger*, Peter Levine describes how animals living in their natural habitats do not suffer from this problem as we humans do; they simply 'wake up', shake out the tension from their bodies and carry on with life (Levine 1997).

We emerge from hypoarousal states first through activation of the sympathetic nervous system, accessing movement again, then returning to social engagement; the first sign might be as small as a deepened breath or a brightening and focusing of the eyes, or it might grow into movement and sound that involve the whole body. Hyperarousal – over-activation of the sympathetic nervous system – needs to be brought into balance through the regulating effect of social engagement with a trusted other, in order for us to feel calm and safe again. In this way, moving up through the evolutionary scale of responses from the vegetative freeze response, through modulation of the fight or flight response, to the social engagement system, the nervous system can return to balanced alignment, and healthy relationship between inner and outer worlds, self and other, can be restored. In somatic work we pay attention to this progression, seeking to restore a client to positive social engagement after work that might have touched layers of traumatic memory with its accompanying physiological and psychological responses.

Holding and Being Held

Over the first year and a half of life after birth, the infant gradually learns to regulate her own autonomic nervous system. The process of primal repression rests upon this, whereby the powerful energies, impulses, images and affects of the Dynamic Ground are quietened. On a basis of good enough care and social engagement, her brain can develop in a healthy way. The process of learning to regulate the autonomic nervous system is mediated by the right hemisphere of the brain, which is associated with sensory, spatial and emotional functions; it is more closely connected with sub-cortical areas of the brain, with the body and with emotional and instinctual behaviours. Right hemisphere attunement between infant and caregiver helps the little one learn to self-regulate and develop a healthy core self (Cozolino 2006: 84).

She first cultivates the capacity to regulate arousal of her sympathetic nervous system; this takes place between 10-14 months. Then regulation of the parasympathetic nervous system follows, from about 14-18 months of age. By the middle of her second year, if all goes well, she has largely mastered the capacity to self-regulate her autonomic nervous system through the process of co-regulation which has been facilitated by her caregivers. Capacities such as self-soothing, calming and being able to wait for something she desires have become possible; good enough attunement and care enable secure attachment behaviours to unfold. Of course, ambivalent, neglectful or abusive care will impede this development and create insecure attachment styles; much has been written about this in the psychological literature (e.g. Cozolino 2006: 139). As we explored earlier, the seeds of attachment styles may have already been sown *in utero* during the stages of conception, implantation and embryological development, and are further elaborated and reinforced during the early months of life.

In order for these crucial developments to take place, the infant needs to be held within the loving and attentive embrace of her caregivers, held with enough sense of boundaries to feel safe and secure, and enough spaciousness to allow for play, learning and growing autonomy. She needs to feel seen as a unique being, not a projection of her parents' desires, expectations or fears. We saw earlier how one of the first tasks of the pre-embryo is the creation of a protective membrane, a containing boundary, within which growth can begin. The middle layer of this membrane, the chorion, is created from cells that are self-structures. The innermost layer, the amnion, evolves after implantation, also from cells that are self-structures of the pre-embryo. The outer layer of the containing membrane is part of the lining of the mother's womb, the endometrium. The embryo is both *container and contents, holding and held*, and this dynamic is expressed most clearly and explicitly in the embryonic formation of this three-layered membrane.

As regulation of the autonomic nervous system and emergence from the Dynamic Ground proceeds, the infant is learning to re-embody at a complex level, and in relationship to others, this miracle of being both held and the one holding. She is learning to hold herself psychologically, with support from caring and attuned others; through the process of co-regulation, her maturing nervous system will enable her to contain much of the anxiety and distress, as well as overwhelming joy and power, which she previously swam within unguarded. To the degree this occurs, the development of the ego can now proceed without too much risk of being overwhelmed by the deep psyche; around five years of age, with the onset of what psychoanalysts call the *latency period*, this is achieved and a new adventure begins.

Part 3

Home and Ground

9: Body as Resource and Healing

The Grounding of Spirit in the Body

In the next two chapters we will explore some of the ways that embodied awareness practices can support us in times when we risk being overwhelmed by powerful energies and emotions arising from the deep psyche. Authentic Movement, and somatic movement practices such as developmental movement therapy, offer potent resources when traumatic material has been activated, or we are touched by energies that move us and move through us – when we are touched by Spirit. As we will see, trauma and the transpersonal live close to each other and both can threaten our stability when we are not grounded in embodied presence.

Marion Woodman writes: "The grounding of the life force in the lowest chakra has to be secure, open to the energies of the earth, before the radiance of the spirit can take up residence." (Woodman 1990: 40) These words feel so wise and true. For the infant, the task of grounding Spirit in the physicality of the body, and in relationship to Earth, involves the extraordinarily hard work of learning to stand and walk. The result is a body that is integrated, powerful and capable of amazing things, and a body-ego that will support further psychological, social and mental development to unfold. The force of pure energy of the Dynamic Ground is channelled through the movement expressions of the infant, toddler and young child. His joy, exuberance, frustration, terror, passion and love become tangible expressions, visible, audible and fully embodied.

During the first months and years of life the maturing of the nervous system both enables and is supported by movement – by the infant's developing capacity to master his own body in relation to the challenges that gravity presents and the needs and desires that are arising in him. Each infant, providing there are no significant neurological challenges (and of course sometimes there sadly are), will progress through a series of movement potentials – *developmental movement patterns* – which are inherent within the nervous system, common to all humans and also to other forms of animate life (Bainbridge Cohen 2018; Hartley 1995; Stokes 2002).

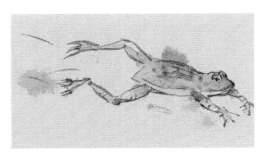
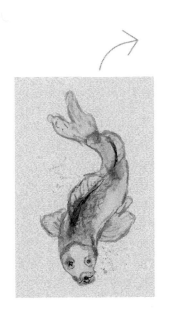
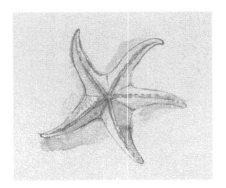

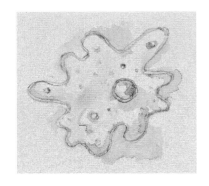

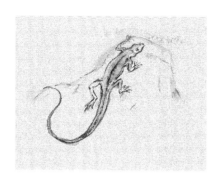

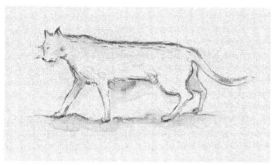

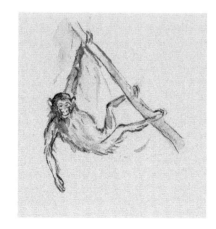

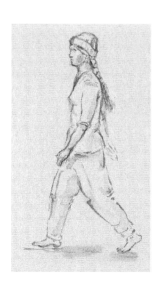

Figures 9.1-9.8: Evolution of movement – Amoeba to Human. Artist: Raima Drąsutytė

Chapter 9: Body as Resource and Healing | 137

First, the original one cell makes *amoeba*-like movement; then, as many cells differentiate out of the one, together they express a *sponge*-like motion as the embryo is forming. The developing foetus and newborn will organise movement around the navel, where the umbilical cord originates, like a *starfish* with limbs radiating out from a mouth at the centre.

During birth we see the emergence of the spinal patterns that a *caterpillar* demonstrates, or a *fish*. On land now, our little one will soon learn to move like an amphibian, such as a *frog*, as he co-ordinates upper limbs and lower limbs to move simultaneously in the homologous pattern; this enables him to bring his head up into the vertical position while lying on his belly, where he can look at the world from a new perspective and discover ways to move out into that world.

He will then go through a phase of very active crawling, using the homolateral pattern that we see in *reptiles* such as salamanders; this allows him to move across the floor with more agency as well as spiral up to a sitting position.

The mature contralateral pattern of *four-legged mammals* finally emerges; this will soon support him, through the brachiation pattern, to move like a *primate*, reaching with his hand for support as he pulls himself up to stand on his two feet.

The journey of learning to walk in *human* fashion depends on and integrates all of these species-typical ways of moving the body through space and up out of gravity. It also integrates the polarities of centre and periphery, upper and lower, back and front, left and right, that were first encountered in the embryological unfolding.

All species are within us; we know them through our embodied movement. When we practise these movement patterns as adults we can sense and feel and see the world from the perspective of our fellow creatures, as well as from the experience of the young infant within us. We are not separate from them, or from our inner child.

As he meets successive challenges and masters ever more complex levels of neuromuscular organisation, the little one is developing muscular strength and co-ordination, skeletal alignment, and tone within organs, nervous system and voice. He is also grounding Spirit within his body so that Spirit becomes immanent, an inherent aspect of embodied being.

This means that his connection to Spirit is both immediate and ever-present, and also increasingly hidden from him as his developing consciousness must engage fully with the changing demands of the material and social realities that confront him at every moment. He is both a pure embodiment of Spirit and a profound expression of bodily existence on Earth. Watch an infant or young child happily at play, or discovering, or relating to an engaged parent and I think you will see what I mean.

As Washburn describes, the source of this energy in the Dynamic Ground will gradually become more hidden, more contained, as primal repression completes. The little one now stands at the threshold of childhood with new tasks to confront, school to attend and social skills to learn as he develops peer relationships outside of his immediate family. Of course, the connection to Spirit is not lost but to some degree it seems to hide from view for a time, until the spiral of growth, or unexpected events, cause its resurgence.

Trauma and the Upsurging of the Deep Psyche

As mentioned earlier, there are natural phases of development when the raw energies of the Dynamic Ground surge back into expression; puberty and adolescence is a time when this happens for every child, as the transition towards adulthood is made. Aside from this, at any point on the arc of development events can so thoroughly overwhelm our capacity to contain feelings and responses that we become traumatised. Unable to integrate the event(s) within the framework of knowing and the capacity to process that have been developed by our ego and our nervous system, we are swept up again in the undercurrents of the deep psyche. The veil is ruptured, the floodgates open, and a too-fragile sense of self can be fragmented by the power of raw, unmitigated life force surging through us. What Winnicott named the 'primitive agonies' of the infant (Davis and Wallbridge 1981: 58) re-surface; the world is experienced once again as Bad Mother, and feelings of terror, aloneness and helplessness are re-activated.

At such times we have moved closer, once again, to unmediated Spirit. At a time when we are at our most vulnerable, most hurt and opened up, our ego defences breached, we are also closest to the core of Spirit that is our Source and ultimate sustenance. Trauma, when we are able to work through it safely, also holds the promise of a deepening to spiritual life.

Experiences of disintegration caused by traumatic events, and the dissolving of the 'small self' during spiritual or mystical experience can live very close to one another. Many mystics as well as psychotherapists recognise this kinship, and the fine line that divides psychosis from spiritual awakening is one that must be attended to with great care in both therapeutic and spiritual practice[1]. In both cases the container of body-ego structures is ruptured, expanded, dissolved or altered in some other way, and that which exists before, beneath and beyond is laid bare. We are immersed, wholly or partially, in the unboundaried, the collective, the Universal.

Referring to the work of Roland Fischer, Peter Levine writes:

> *[I]t appears that the very brain structures that are central to the resolution of trauma are also pivotal in various "mystical" and "spiritual" states.*
>
> *In the East, the awakening of Kundalini at the first (or survival) chakra center has long been known to be a vehicle for initiating ecstatic transformation. In trauma, a similar activation is provoked, but with such intensity and rapidity that it overwhelms the organism. If we can gradually access and integrate this energy into our nervous system and psychic structures, then the survival response embedded within trauma can also catalyze authentic spiritual transformation.* (Levine 2010: 350)

Janet Adler has noted the similarity between trauma and mystical experience in movement expressions that arise in the Discipline of Authentic Movement. Gestures and movement patterns which emerge and develop during the exploration and resolution of traumatic material eventually transform, as the charge of energy bound up in the trauma is expressed, compassionately witnessed and integrated over time; we then discover the same gestures arising, but now the experience is of a transpersonal or mystical nature – an awakening to a world of coherent body infused with numinous Spirit, of self at one with the Universal:

> *It is not uncommon for a gesture that forms within a body memory of a trauma to become the gesture which marks the gateway into transpersonal experiences.* (Adler 2002: 232)

Trauma can occur at any stage of life. As some therapists working with pre- and peri-natal processes have noted, even pre-conception can be a vulnerable time for the soul entering embodied life (Castellino 1995). Conception and any point along the embryological journey pose challenges and risks. Implantation is a particularly significant moment, when the new being is called to make the commitment to embed in *this* body, with *this* mother, and embrace the path of incarnation in *this* particular life. At each step a new challenge arises; if inner readiness is not aligned with outer support, acceptance and love, then disruption can occur.

Healing through Movement and Embodied Awareness

Because somatic movement practice and the Discipline of Authentic Movement support the integration of body and mind, soma and psyche, they can help cultivate a coherent and integrated container for the powerful energies of the deep psyche and Spirit. Embodied awareness practice offers many resources for the healing of trauma and other imbalances, stresses and disruptions within us. Without a secure container of embodied presence, the full processing of trauma, which is as much a physiological as a psychological condition, cannot happen. And without embodied awareness, the path towards healing trauma might be less safely embarked upon. Keeping awareness rooted in the body, we are better able to stay present as we confront overwhelming feelings, powerful energies and disturbing sensations[2].

In post-traumatic stress disorder, an historic traumatic event is re-activated, triggered by something in the present situation which shares some element in common with the original trauma; it is felt to be still occurring, in the present moment, even though it might have happened long ago. The same neurological and chemical pathways that were laid down during the original trauma are re-activated, so that the body itself tells us that we are still experiencing the threat or danger. Sweating palms, heart palpitations, fast and erratic breathing patterns, dizziness and feelings of nausea are some of the signs; there may be the paralysing weakness of hypoarousal if the vegetative parasympathetic nervous system has been activated, or uncontrolled expressions of rage and panic if hyperarousal of the sympathetic nervous system is occurring. Repeated flashbacks and nightmares are common.

It is hard to escape this cycle of physiological and psychological symptoms without external support. We have lost contact with the present moment, with the here-and-now of our bodily existence, and this must be restored in order for post-traumatic stress to be managed, released and integrated into *post-traumatic learning*. This needs to happen in a safe relational context, as lack of this was likely part of the original situation.

Somatic trauma therapies recognise the need and the value of discovering and applying *resources* that can reverse the negative cycle of triggers and symptoms of post-traumatic stress disorder (Rothschild 2000). When we engage in, or even think about and immerse ourselves in, the memory and sensations of something that generates positive feelings, we experience a whole body-mind shift away from the re-activated trauma response towards balance. Like the re-activation of the trauma itself, the re-balancing is both physiological and psychological – as our mental state transforms through positive memory or image, so does the physiology and chemistry of the body, and we can step away from the state of hyperarousal or hypoarousal that has been triggered. Once resourced and in balance again, we can return to the distressing event(s) and symptoms to explore and release the next layer of bound up energy.

To resolve traumatic experiences our brain needs to be able to locate the event(s) clearly in the past and recognise that here and now, in this current moment and situation, we are safe. When this recognition can be fully embraced the body and mind can return to balance and presence.

The Discipline of Authentic Movement

Peter Levine developed the model of SIBAM for the resolution of trauma through working with the body. This stands for Sensation – Image – Behaviour – Affect – Meaning, all of which need to be incorporated into safe and effective trauma work (Levine 2010: 139). In the Discipline of Authentic Movement we follow a similar path. First, we ground the movement experience in the body by tracking the movements (behaviour), gestures and arising sensations; we continually return to this ground as we speak about our experience as mover or witness. If we are aware of sensation and movement (through the kinaesthetic sense) we can be nowhere other than in the present moment, in this body, this time and place. We return to presence each time we are able to witness our movement and sensations. In this way, Authentic Movement can offer a safe ground for opening to emotionally distressing or traumatic material that might surface from unconscious layers of the psyche during movement practice.

Upon this ground we layer our awareness of all we are feeling (affect) during the movement time, as mover or witness, and as we speak about it afterwards. The faintest hint of a feeling or the most insistent and loud expression of emotion – all is embraced, given space, allowed to express to the extent that this can be done safely. This safety is supported by the tracking of where the body is, how we are moving and the accompanying sensations.

If image or story arises, this too can be named. Here we are careful not to use image as an easy way to label our experience – "I have an image of a tiger" – and leave it at that. An image can serve as a portal into the full knowing of the depth and breadth of our experience in that moment. We want to know more: we describe the movement in detail to discover what about the movement suggests tiger; and open to the sensations and feelings that are present so that we come to know the essence of tiger as it exists in our own embodied being. My experience of tiger-ness might be very different from yours; the details of movement, sensation, feeling and energy help us to reach into the essence and source of our experience in that moment.

This in turn can lead to insight, a spontaneous discovery of meaning. In the Discipline of Authentic Movement we refrain from using analysis and interpretation, but allow insight and meaning to arise out of the practice of awareness, within the mover's own timing and readiness. This allows for a deepening of the movement material, which can lead to unexpected and as-yet-unknown places being uncovered. We seek to arrive at the essence of the movement experience, which leads the mover to a deepened connection to herself and her intuitive knowing.[3]

In a similar way meditation practice invites a non-analytical approach that can open us to insight and intuitive knowing. Thich Nhat Hanh writes:

> *Understanding should not be only empty knowledge, but deep insight. Insight is not the outcome of thinking. Insight is a kind of direct intuitive vision that you get from strong concentration. It's not a product of thinking. It is a deep intuition. And, if it is a real insight, it will have the power to free you from your anger, your fear, your suffering.* (Thich Nhat Hanh 2021: 18)

Over time and many hours of practice, the energetic charge held within unconscious (not-yet-known) or traumatic material can be safely expressed and integrated into consciousness, held within the container that is created by the witness's presence and awareness, and the mover's own evolving inner witness. As the traumatic material resolves, sometimes the same gestures that held the trauma might re-appear to reveal the phenomenon of pure energy moving through the body. The mystery of Spirit, the Numinous, may be glimpsed or experienced in its fullness.

Developmental Movement Therapy

These skills and processes are brought to bear within somatic movement therapy. One foundation of the practice I work with and have taught extensively, rooted in Body-Mind Centering, is the sequence of *developmental movement patterns*, briefly outlined above, which the new being embarks upon before, during and after birth. I and others have written about this work more fully elsewhere, so I give only brief descriptions here (See Bainbridge Cohen 2008, 2018; Hartley 1995, 2004; Stokes 2002). Each of these movement processes enables the embodiment of certain qualities that can be resourcing for the person learning to heal from trauma, or experiencing directly the phenomenon of energy in the body when entering the realm of mystical practice. I name a few here and invite you to try some of the examples; they might be familiar to you from previous study and practice, or this may be a new area of practice.

If you wish to try these practices, I suggest taking one theme at a time and exploring this until it feels comfortable and natural to you before moving on to the next. Notice how they change your state of being and feeling, and might be resourcing. I offer potential qualities that might be experienced, though it is more useful that you discover your own connections. Or you might prefer to simply read the introductions and resources and maybe put time aside later to try out the movement practices.

Cellular Breathing

The internal respiration of cells is the first movement of embodied life and an ever-present subtle motion throughout our whole lifetime. Each cell pulses, expanding as fluid, oxygen and nutritional molecules are absorbed into the cell; condensing as the cell releases wastes, along with molecular messengers that will communicate with other cells of the body.

> ➢ Placing a hand very lightly over any part of your body which calls for attention, sense the skin of your palm and fingers meeting the skin of the body part (directly or through clothing). Rest here for a moment and settle into the touch.
>
> ➢ Imagine one cell, or a group of cells that lie beneath your hand. Visualise the cellular membrane, containing a fluid cytoplasmic body, a nucleus

that is home to the DNA, and many organelles that carry out the cell's vital functions, just as organs do for the body as a whole.

- ➤ Simply rest here and breathe, connecting to the presence of the cell(s) and the subtle pulse of cellular breathing, which is considerably quicker than external breathing. Allow each cell to take up its space in the body and breathe more fully; invite each cell to feel its own relationship to the Earth and yield its delicate weight into gravity.

- ➤ You might get a sense of the quality of containment that the cell membrane gives. You might become aware of how you feel and the quality of attention that this practice brings. Receive and enjoy whatever arises.

RESOURCE: This practice can bring feelings of peace, wholeness and simply Being, offering a foundation for experiencing embodied presence as well as nurturing rest and recuperation. It is a practice that invites us to attend, to listen inwardly and receive the embodied wisdom within us.

Navel Radiation

In utero the embryo develops an umbilical cord and placenta that serve to nourish the foetus throughout gestation. The navel, where the umbilical cord extends from the body, serves as a centre of organisation, not only for the passage of nutrients and wastes in and out of the body but also a centre around which early movement is organised. This pattern is also visible in the newborn where we see the limbs – upper spine to the head and face, tail of the spine and pelvic floor, two arms and two legs – involved in a dance with each other through the navel centre. The foetus, and later the newborn, explores movement potentials as she flexes and extends her limbs, curls into her centre and opens out to touch the boundaries of her womb-home.

- ➤ Find a comfortable place to lie down on your back, or your belly if you prefer, with your arms and legs gently spread out and resting on the floor; release your weight into the ground and breathe for a few moments.

➤ Imagine your breath is entering and leaving your body through your navel, filling and emptying the middle of your body first. Let it slow and deepen, and begin to imagine that as you take a breath in it spreads from the navel gradually along all of your six limbs, out towards the head and tail, tips of fingers and toes. As you breathe out the breath returns to the navel and is released. Allow your whole body to fill and empty with the breath.

➤ Begin to allow a little movement through your six limbs. You can start with just one or two, or all limbs moving together, whatever feels most easeful. As you breathe in and fill, allow a lengthening, expanding, extending, reaching outwards. As you breathe out and empty, allow your limbs to soften, flex, fold back in towards your centre.

➤ The movements can be very small and subtle at first, then allow them to grow as you play with folding and unfolding, flexing and extending, gathering in to yourself and opening out to the world. Sometimes two or more limbs move towards and away from each other; sometimes all limbs move together. There are limitless possibilities. Explore as if discovering movement for the first time.

➤ Feel the dance of relationship between your centre and the endpoints of your six limbs as each part comes to know each other part through the centre. (This is a lovely thing to do when you first wake up in the morning, a way to gently ready yourself to get out of bed and start your day.)

RESOURCE: This pattern enables us to feel the body as many distinct parts but also one integrated whole; the experience of being many parts that are all in relationship with and connected to each other through the centre supports the *invariant of coherency*, vital for the emergence of a sense of *core self*, as Stern describes (Stern 1985: 82).

This pattern also provides a foundation for alternating movement inwards, towards self and centre, and outwards, to others and the world beyond; we will be challenged to balance these two movements throughout life. When we explore the *navel radiation pattern* we might discover where we are within this inner-outer cycle right now, and what support we need to continue the healthy dance of alternating between them.

Spinal Patterns

Early in the development of the embryo we see the emergence of an axis through the length of the body, first expressed as the *notochord*, then the spinal cord, digestive tube and vertebral spine begin to grow. Birth evokes the full embodiment of movements that flow along the length of the spine, from head to tail and tail to head, as the spine and its supporting structures integrate to form a central core. First the birthing child engages in pushing her way through the birth canal; then, at the moment of release, her head pulls her whole body out and into a new world of air, gravity and other.

- Come to the 'baby posture' on the floor or a mattress: kneel with knees spread, toes touching, and lower your forehead to the ground (using a cushion if you wish); let your elbows widen out to each side and your hands rest on the floor above your head, fingertips touching. Take a few moments to release and breathe as your body settles into this place. (Adapt the posture to suit your own body if it is not comfortable.)

- Gently rock your body forwards so that you come up onto the crown of your head, rolling over the surface of your cranium. Rest here for a moment, releasing as much weight as is comfortable through the top of your head into the Earth, your forearms taking the rest of the weight.

- Gently rock back onto your heels, rolling over the surface of your cranium so that your head stays in contact with the floor throughout.

- Repeat this as often as you like. Gradually begin to feel the gentle *push* against the ground which initiates the movement – pushing from the front of the feet and the tail of the spine as you rock forwards; from the crown of your head as you rock back.

- Connect with the sense of movement flowing up and down along your spine throughout the movement, connecting head and tail.

- Come back to your heels, unroll your spine and feel your verticality, supported by a clear sense of your spine at the core of your body. Can you feel a lift or reach upwards through the top of your head and a reach down into the Earth from your tail? This subtle feeling holds the potential to initiate movements that open out into the space beyond your head and tail, drawing you out and beyond your own boundaries.

RESOURCE:
These movements, which gently mirror the movements of birth, can help us to feel the core structures of our spine, creating a sense of vertical support and underlying the *sense of core self* (Stern 1985: 69). They support our feeling of connection to both the Earth beneath us and Heaven above, aligned and connected through our own body.

Yield and Push

To further explore the action of pushing which was introduced in the *spinal patterns*, I now invite you to experience active *yielding*. This prepares for the pushing, reaching and pulling actions that initiate the infant's journey towards full-bodied exploration of space.

> ➢ This can be done from any position – standing, sitting, lying down or wherever you find yourself to be. Take a moment to connect to the surfaces of your body that touch the ground, whether this is the floor surface, the bare earth, a chair, cushion or mattress. Allow your mind to move through these places of contact. How fully can you release the weight of your body into the support that is offered?

> ➢ *Yielding* is not a passive state, which can lead to inertia and immobility. It is an active engagement of the mind and the body's weight with the supporting surface, ultimately with the Earth.

> ➢ Feel the movement of mind, cells, fluids and body weight towards the centre of the Earth. After a while you will feel a response – an impulse, an energy, a subtle force rising to meet you through the place of contact. Allow your body to respond to this impulse: you might lengthen and slide or roll along the floor, or you might begin the journey of rising up out of the floor. An easeful *pushing* movement orients around the place of contact; keep your mind focused here as each shift allows another meeting place, another moment of yielding and being moved by the Earth in response. Allow the dialogue between body and Earth to unfold.

> ➢ *Yield and Push* can initiate movement through the whole body at any point of contact with the ground. Often it is a hand or foot, a knee or an elbow; in the *spinal patterns* it is the head or tail of the spine but it could be the ribs, the side of the pelvis, the outer surface of the

arm or any other place. Allow yourself to yield through whichever part of your body is meeting the ground and feel the energy of the Earth rising up through that place and into you, initiating movement across the floor or upwards and through the space. Allow yourself to discover new movements.

RESOURCE:
Yielding invites us to come into intimate contact with the Earth beneath us or another supporting surface that mediates that connection; for the infant this is first of all her mother's body, which is Earth and ground to her. It allows us to feel the depth of support which being in embodied relationship with the Earth can give us. An attitude of respectful and receptive listening, attending to and loving Earth might evolve from this.

You might come to feel that you are a conscious moving aspect of the Earth expressing herself, the Earth dancing herself into conscious awareness.

Pushing into and out of the ground strengthens the sense of body boundaries, the sense of self, of having strength, power and agency, of being an integrated whole; it can resource us when we feel overwhelmed, fragmented, disoriented or disconnected.

Reach and Pull

There is a natural continuum from *yield and push* to *reach and pull*. As the yield supports a push and the impulse travels through the body, another endpoint of the body will be supported to reach out into space. For example, if the infant is lying on her belly and finds her right foot pushing against the floor so that the whole right side of her body extends and is lengthened headwards, the movement completes in the reaching of her right hand forwards. She has initiated a movement of homolateral crawling.

If there is impetus and desire – the desire to touch or grab hold of something or someone over there, just beyond reach – the infant will reach out a hand to pull herself towards the object of her interest. Desire, intention, agency and will come together as a *reach* beyond the 'known and safe' is supported, and she can *pull* herself towards that which lies 'just beyond'.

➢ After exploring *yield and push* for a while, notice when an impulse has travelled through your body and begins to initiate a *reach* into space, upwards or across the floor, or perhaps across your body to create turning or spiralling pathways.

> Without forcing yourself to go further than is easy and right for you in this moment, notice when the energy builds so that the *reach* becomes more active, focused and directed; allow the capacity to *pull* your whole body through space from one of your extremities (head/face/senses, tail of spine/pelvic floor, fingertips, toes) to emerge naturally from this. Your senses, especially your vision but also your ears, nose and tongue will support you in this.

RESOURCE:
When we have yielded into the Earth to find support, discovered the capacity to push with both ease and power from this supportive ground, strengthening our sense of self, grounding and personal boundaries, we are ready to relate to others and the world around us in more diverse and articulate ways. Practising movements that we initiate with a *reach and pull* enables us to explore and develop the capacity and the courage to reach beyond our known boundaries and limits for what we desire and need, to explore and discover; we learn to orient to the world around us and come into relationship in ways that feel right, supported by our conscious awareness of self and other. *Social engagement* is enabled by this capacity.

These resources offer embodied grounding that can support us to more safely encounter trauma and strong emotional charge in the body. Energetic phenomena that might arise when Spirit moves us, and moves through us, can also be more securely surrendered to when psyche and soma are well-integrated through such practices. We can practise during times of calm so that resources are more readily available when the need arises.

10: Supporting Presence in Relationship

Meeting the world is a relational dance at the heart of the infant's journey into embodied life. It is also at the heart of, and not separate from, the impulse to touch and be touched by Spirit. The dance of embodying Spirit involves deepening connection with self, with others, with the more-than-human world and the mysterious Source of all of life. The impulse to surrender to, dissolve into and be transformed by Spirit lives in us with equal measure of fear and longing. We need inner resources, courage and determination to pursue this path. To come into relationship with Spirit and become at-one with the Universal is the ultimate quest of the authentic mystic and seeker of embodied spirituality. It comes from a place of deepened connection with self, from where we may begin to open to ever-expanding layers of connectedness.

The dance of opening inwardly towards self and opening outwardly towards other is the beating pulse of our embodied life. With each beat the heart draws blood into its empty chambers, holds it there for a moment of stillness and rest, then releases it out and around the whole body. In, out. As with the breath, incoming followed by outgoing breath in endless alternation. Whilst heart and breath keep their work going without our conscious intervention, to navigate the dance of relationship throughout our lives requires care, attention, inner and outer listening, and reliable resources. The *embodied relational spiritual practice* that is offered through somatic movement and the Discipline of Authentic Movement can support this journey, bringing consciousness to the dynamics of inner and outer connection.

Merete Brantbjerg, a Danish therapist specialising in relational trauma therapy[1], has developed a protocol for connecting to self and other when working with trauma. She calls it Resource Oriented Skills Training (ROST). The sequence of skills can be practised by therapists as support for their work with clients, as well as by the clients themselves as a way of learning to resource themselves through embodied practice. They are also helpful to any of us wanting to stay grounded and connected as we open out to widening circles of relationship in our lives, and in those rarer moments when we are graced with the presence of Spirit.

I find that this simple protocol closely follows the developmental movement sequence, briefly outlined in the last chapter. Below are the six skills that Brantbjerg describes, and a brief description of how somatic practice and developmental movement processes might support and enrich them (with thanks to Merete Brantbjerg for the clarity of this sequence):

Grounding

> This skill is essential in work with traumatised clients, as with anyone in distress, emotionally charged or disoriented. We need to know where we stand and what supports us before we can begin to move through the difficulty. One of Bonnie Bainbridge Cohen's maxims is 'support before movement', as mentioned earlier; grounding is an essential way in which we find this support.

> The practice of *yielding into* and *pushing out of* the Earth is a way to enter this process. In my own teaching of this sequence, I would invite students to include the body systems which most support them to find grounding: for many it is feeling the transfer of weight down through the bones; for some, the skin contacting the floor or the muscles pushing against it; or releasing the weight of the organs into gravity. They are invited to explore the yielding of weight *into* the floor and pushing *out of* the floor to find *grounding down* and *grounding up* respectively.

Flexibility

> If we only ground we might begin to feel too earth-bound, solid and immobile, so we need to remember our flexibility and fluidity too. We find this in the joints of the skeletal system, together with the muscles that enable the bones to move around the joints. And in all the different fluids of the body, each of which brings its own quality, rhythm and flow of movement. Flowing, streaming, jiggling, sustained or dynamic fluid motion is encouraged as an opening of all the joints of the body, head to toes, centre to periphery, is explored. Fluid movement through the whole body invites a gentle loosening of the mind's control and the expression of many different qualities of expression.

Centering

Somatic work offers many ways to find and move from or around our centre. There are different centres in the body that we can explore – the head, heart, solar plexus, Hara or Tan Tien, spine and vertical axis, the centre of gravity. Some practitioners may work with others. For the purpose of this exploration, we consider the area at the front of the mid-lumbar spine, close to the centre of gravity and Tan Tien or Hara, to be the centre. It is also close to the navel so the navel radiation pattern can be felt as a support. Movements which balance around the centre help to stimulate the deep core muscles in this region, strengthening balance and integration. Trauma and damage to the sense of core self might reflect in difficulty as these movements are practised.

The movement pattern which most clearly activates this area is the *contralateral* pattern, our most developmentally evolved co-ordination that integrates all dimensions as we crawl, walk or run. As right arm and left leg, left arm and right leg, work together, muscles around the centre of the body are activated to maintain balance and co-ordinated whole-body movement. This pattern stimulates all muscles of the body as sagittal, vertical and horizontal dimensions are integrated in spirallic movement forms. Simply walking is one of the most profound and well-used ways to cultivate internal integration, connection and centring. In fact walking, by the sea or in the woods if possible, is recommended by trauma therapists as being especially resourcing and healing.

Boundaries

Once we have grounded, recovered our fluidity and flexibility, and centred ourselves, we can begin to look out towards connection and relationship. The first stage is to affirm our personal boundaries. Our skin, as primary boundary, can be awakened through focusing awareness within it as we move, and through touch – the touch of our own hands, stroking, pinching, tapping, etc; or contact with the floor, wall and other surfaces. Then we extend our awareness to fill our *kinosphere*, the personal space that surrounds us and into which we can reach and extend ourselves. It is usually felt to extend as far as we can reach with our limbs; I believe it mirrors and may be an energetic imprint of our first container, the amniotic sac in which we spent our pre-natal life.

Extending our limbs to define this space, filling it with our movement and our attention, we take up the space that is ours and allow ourselves to feel the fullness of presence that this brings.

Orienting in Space

As with the infant who has mastered the yield and push initiations and is ready to go beyond his personal sphere, we now look, listen, sense and feel into the wider space around us and begin to orient to it: where do I want to be within this space, in relation to others? How do I want to move in relation to the space and others? This is supported by our externally-oriented senses, just as the infant's adventures into an ever-widening world are supported by his curiosity and his awakened senses. Sometimes we might be called to *reach and pull* ourselves beyond the safe and known boundaries of our personal space.

This naturally takes us to the last skill – negotiating right relationship.

Negotiating Relationship

If we do not feel grounded and centred, have lost the feeling of flexibility that would allow us to adjust and respond, and are not clear within our own body boundaries and sense of self, we will find the tasks of orienting to where we need to be in space and negotiating relationship with others challenging. If these skills are embodied well enough, we can open to relationship in ways that respect both our own needs, wishes and feelings, and those of the other in appropriate measure. A sense of rightness in relationship can be more easily created, and the damage that inability to access these resources so often engenders, can be lessened.

I invite you to explore these skills, finding the movements and the sources of movement that best support you to engage with each. They should be practised as a sequence, moving organically to the next stage once you feel secure within each one (grounding and flexibility can be interchanged – start where you most feel the need or the readiness to engage). The overall intention is to first connect to your own embodied self so that you feel present; then you are ready to open out to the world and others from this place, supported to maintain presence as you engage and interact. You can explore this sequence with music of your choice if you like, and with other movers if possible.

Balancing the Autonomic Nervous System

The body's physiology reflects many ways of supporting and regulating the balance between inner and outer, our own needs and the demands of our environment. This dynamic balance is embedded deeply into our cells, fluids and tissues. Present in each breath and each heartbeat, in the cycles of the autonomic nervous system, in every step we take, we seek equilibrium from moment to moment as we oscillate around the centre of balance. Problems can occur when these oscillations are disrupted, when we become stuck at some point, or one side comes to dominate.

Sensory-motor processing – the feedback loops between information coming in and information going out – enables the infant's movement potentials to unfold, and on this foundation a clear sense of self and healthy ego structure can develop. Spirit becomes embodied within the cells, bones, muscles and viscera of the growing child, grounded within the body. The sequence of movement development outlined in the last chapter, and the resource skills that reflect the essence of this development, support the emergence of a healthy and integrated soma-psyche that is capable of 'holding' Spirit until it is ready to reveal itself again.

Within a 'good enough' environment, a healthy relationship to self and others can grow, and upon this foundation emotional, social, mental and spiritual development can unfold. As we have seen, the dynamic between inner and outer, self and other, is a core concern from the embryonic beginnings of life. It continues to be central to the infant's development throughout the first months and years of life. Balancing inner needs and desires with the needs and demands of those we come into relationship with requires ongoing attention. Good enough nurturing and care in infancy and early childhood gifts the child with the resources needed to manage this delicate balancing act. The child who has been supported to regulate their autonomic nervous system develops the capacity to embody health-giving cycles of rest and activity, alternating periods of outgoing challenge with incoming recuperation. They can regulate the relationship between outer and inner, opening out to the world and returning inwards to self when needed.

When there has been trauma, this can be followed by disruption in the natural progress of development and a fracturing of the sense of core self. Natural and healthy cycles within the autonomic nervous system are disturbed: it can be difficult to calm, ground, centre within oneself and receive nurturing; the challenges that life poses might feel impossible to navigate, and chaos and disorder ensue, instead of contentment and fulfilment.

Many physiological, psychological and social symptoms result from difficulties in meeting and balancing our inner needs with outer circumstances and demands. The relationship between inner and outer, our interior life and the world we inhabit, is disturbed. A multitude of social, historical, global and environmental factors inevitably play a part in this, impacting all of us in complex ways; they cannot be separated from the issues a traumatised individual must confront.

Much has been written in the psychological and neuroscientific literature about the complex symptoms of, and pathways towards, healing personal and collective trauma. It is not my intention to add to this here. My focus is towards embodied practices and how they can help us to navigate our way through these complexities through cultivating embodied presence. Turning to somatic therapies is one way to begin to return to more healthful cycles within the autonomic nervous system (see for example Okondo, in Hartley 2022: Ch 15). Several ways in which our body and innate movement potentials support the balance of the autonomic nervous system have already been mentioned. Here I review some of these and outline how they are built upon as the complexity of a growing human being evolves. (Some of the movements and practices described below are complex in their detail and some readers might want to skip these examples for now, perhaps creating space later to dive in more deeply; if you are interested to explore further you might like to seek out a practitioner who can guide you in more specific ways[3].)

Inside and Outside – the Cell

From the beginning the cell membrane serves as an interface and primary boundary between self and other. The process of cellular breathing, or internal respiration, carries nutrition and information between the interior of the cell and its environment. This offers a template for the lifelong work of balancing the capacity to receive and to give, to take in what we need and to release what we no longer need or might be needed by others. Right relationship begins at the membrane of the cell.

Cellular Membrane – an Enquiry:

The practice of connecting to and enquiring into the condition of my cellular membranes is one I can engage with in different ways – I might take time, lying or sitting comfortably, relaxing and allowing my mind to settle into the presence of cells breathing. This happens below the threshold of everyday awareness, but can be accessed when I take time to stop and listen inwardly. Once this practice is familiar, I may be able to connect instantaneously to the presence of cells and their membranes when I bring my attention there.

The cell membrane is a double-layered molecular structure that faces both inwards to the interior of the cell and outwards to the external ocean of interstitial fluid. I visualise, sense, feel and embody this presence within me. As it becomes clearer, I enquire: how does the membrane, as interface between inside and outside, feel? What quality of containment does it offer – is it a semi-permeable membrane that allows the passage of fluids through? Or is it too rigid, too permeable or damaged in some way? Too thick or too thin, or with gaps and tears? At different times, and in different parts of my body, it might be any of these.

I also want to know: do the cells communicate with each other or do they seem to work in isolation? I notice that, at different times in my life, the answer to this question might change, depending on how I am feeling and what circumstances I find myself in. The condition of the cellular membranes can give me valuable information as to what I might need to receive, give, change in my life.

Autonomic Rhythm

As the embryo begins to form, held between the yolk sac at the front (nurturing Mother principle) and the amniotic sac at the back (protective Father principle), a subtle rhythm is established: fluid seeps between the yolk and amniotic sacs through a space, the *neuroenteric canal*, that forms at the centre of the developing embryo's midline. The two sacs alternately fill slightly and empty slightly, and a subtle opening and closing movement occurs in the pre-embryo. It is a long and slow rhythm, slower than external breathing and, as mentioned in chapter 6, is related to the craniosacral *long tide* (Kern 2001: 15) and the *autonomic rhythm*, which underlies the foundational rhythm of the autonomic nervous system (Bainbridge Cohen 2008: 186). When this rhythm flows with ease, gently alternating between opening out and folding back in, there is health and balance within the autonomic nervous system. It flows through all cells of the body, front to back and back to front. We might also feel the integration of Mother and Father archetypal energies if we can surrender to the holding that is offered at this embryonic stage of development by the yolk and amniotic sacs. The following exploration is based on Bonnie Bainbridge Cohen's work, a version of which was described earlier; here you can go deeper into the experience if you wish:

Embodying the Yolk and Amniotic Sacs

➢ Standing (or sitting or lying on one side if you prefer), imagine you are the embryonic disc: two-layered, you have a front-body and a back-body. From your front-body, some cells have migrated to form a big (yolk) sac, a fluid-filled cushion in front of you. From your back-body, some cells have migrated to form another big (amniotic) sac, a fluid-filled cushion behind you. You are completely held and supported between the two sacs. Take some time to feel into this total body support.

➢ After a while, if you listen to your body in an attentive and receptive way, you might feel a very subtle impulse to extend, to open and arch your body slightly backwards, not over-extending but buoyant with the felt-sense of cellular fluids moving back; or an impulse to softly curve your body forwards, not collapsing but full and supported as the fluid within the cells seeps forward. Go with this; it can be a very small movement to begin with, little more than an internal feeling of spacious opening and leaning back then a suspended leaning forward as you fill and curve over the fluid-filled sacs at the back and the front.

➢ Listen carefully for the impulse to reverse the direction; take time, there is no need to rush. Wait until there is a clear sense of an impulse to fold in or extend out, to curve or arch.

- ➢ Continue for as long as you wish. Let the movements grow through your whole body if this feels right. You are being moved by the rhythm of fluids flowing between front and back, within each cell; the movement is fluid and easy.

- ➢ Come to rest in standing, feeling the balance between the front and back of your body. Make any small adjustments that are needed to arrive in easeful balance.

Gestures of the Embryo

As we saw earlier, the miracle of embryonic formation resembles a kind of organic origami, a complex folding, enfolding and unfolding of groups of cells as organs and body tissues come into being. We also saw that what was inner moves outwards; what faced out, turns inwards. The gestures of formation speak to this dance between inner and outer so that the two polarities are intimately interwoven; in fact, we can hardly look upon them as two different environments, but rather one continuum that endlessly seeks to renew and reform itself in relation to its dual nature of interior and exterior world. Although we all experience an 'I' that has a sense of being an inner world, the embryo shows us that 'I' is not separate from all that we consider 'other' and outside of us.

Navel Radiation Pattern

As described previously, this radial organisation of movement offers a playground for the foetus and newborn to explore and discover their six limbs in movement, and the relationship of each limb to each other limb through connection to the navel centre. They are also discovering relationship between their own body boundaries, the fluid environment they swim within, and the membranes of the womb that contain them. Limbs can fold in to touch self – toes touching fingers, fingers touching face, they explore and come to know themself. Reaching out, they can swim freely in their own fluid ocean and press, kick or stroke the walls of the womb-world. They are beginning to learn about self and other through this exploratory play.

Deeper In and Further Out

Physiological Flexion and Extension

Embedded in the womb, the material body of the foetus is growing at a remarkable rate, powered by the constant source of nourishment from the mother's body. By the third trimester the foetus is essentially fully formed, all organ systems in place and gradually developing functionality. Now a primary task is to grow in size, weight and strength as she becomes ready for the challenges of birth and life beyond the womb. As she grows, the space inside the womb becomes tighter, more constricted. This stimulates the development of *tone* in the muscles, organs and nervous system.

Tone is the baseline activity of muscle and other tissue when at rest; good tone means the muscle is always ready to act, to respond to changing needs with differing levels of activation. If tone is too high or too low it will be harder to respond with the right amount of strength, speed, precision and control. The constricting embrace of the womb in the later months of gestation stimulates tone, first in the flexor muscles and the organs then, slightly later, in the extensor muscles and the spinal cord. Extensor tone will not be fully expressed until birth, when the infant alternates between flexion and extension, and finally extends fully at the moment of emergence from the birth canal.

The development of *physiological flexion and extension* is a process, not a movement pattern as such, but we can practise an alternating full-body flexion and extension pattern to activate tone throughout the whole body and create balance between flexion and extension, front and back. This evolves out of the embryonic pattern of opening and closing that we saw earlier, but now with the vitality and power of muscular and organic activity. It can feel deeply enjoyable and satisfying to move between being fully flexed, curled in around oneself, and fully extended and open to the world. Interestingly, tone develops first from the toes and feet, proceeding upwards towards the neck; tone of the fingers and hands begins as tone in the hip and pelvic area is developing, also proceeding from periphery to centre.

Exploring Physiological Flexion and Extension

This can be done with a partner who can give feedback through touch as to where the movement is initiating and sequencing through the body, but exploring on your own with clear attention and intention is also excellent practice.

> *Physiological Flexion*: Begin lying on one side, your body gently flexed. Take your attention to your toes and flex your toes under, as deeply as is comfortable, then flex your ankle (up, as if you were standing) at the same time. Try this a few times until it begins to feel natural. This movement is natural for a baby but less familiar for us as adults – imagine you are picking up a pencil from the floor with the sole of your foot to get the feeling of it.

> Let the flexion sequence up both legs, in turn flexing knee then hip. At the same time can you very gently activate the tone in your pelvic organs? Feel that toning, subtly activating the deep pelvic organs, is the impulse for the flexion and drawing up of the toes and feet. It might help to imagine a thread from the pelvic organs to the toes being gently pulled up.

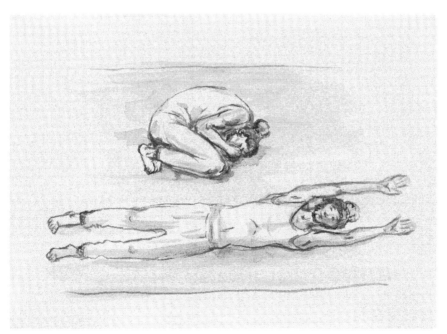

Figure 10.1: Physiological flexion and extension.
Artist: Raima Drąsutytė

- ➢ As your hip joints are flexing, your fingers also begin to curl in, followed by wrists, elbows and shoulders.

- ➢ Now the whole spine is flexing, starting at the tail and moving sequentially up to the neck. Feel that the organs also sequentially increase their tone, initiating or supporting the flexion of the spine from tail to head, as drawing in of the lower limbs proceeds.

- ➢ You will arrive in a tightly flexed foetal position.

- ➢ *Physiological Extension*: Once again begin with toes and ankles, this time reversing the movement at each joint. First the toes extend then the ankles extend (plantar flexion, as if you were standing on your toes). Gradually sequence the extension through knees and hip joints. Can you feel a subtle activation in your spinal cord, beginning at the tail end and sequencing up as you begin to extend your legs?

- ➢ As your hip joints are opening, your fingers also begin to uncurl. Let the extension sequence through wrists, elbows and shoulders until your arms are fully extended along the floor above your head.

- ➢ At the same time your spine is extending, from the tail up towards the neck, and maybe your face, eyes and mouth are opening too.

- ➢ You will arrive in a fully extended and elongated position.

- ➢ Alternate the flexion and extension several times, then roll over and do the same on the other side.

- ➢ Allow yourself to improvise with the feeling of full body extension and flexion – rolling, stretching, curling in, opening out. Notice how you feel in these two gestures of opening out and gathering in.

- ➢ Coming to stand at the end, feel into the relationship between flexor and extensor tone throughout your whole body as you balance around your centre.

Birth

The development of tone prepares the foetus for the momentous journey of birth; she will be called to yield into the increasing pressure from the contracting womb, folding even more deeply into herself, into full-bodied flexion. Here she is gathering the strength and power to push against the contracting walls of the womb and through the birth canal, as she discovers the power of the push that enables her to extend her body. At the moment of birth, as she spirals out of the birth canal, she can finally lengthen into full extension as she enters her new world.

The Support of Primitive Reflexes

As the neuromuscular system develops in complexity, specific reflexive responses begin to emerge out of whole-body flexor and extensor tone. More differentiated movement expressions are evoked by specific stimuli, a call-and-response dialogue between outer environment and inner processing, which enables specific movements to be elicited. Some occur in particular parts of the body; others involve all or most of the body. (I will not go into the full details of these complex responses here but refer the interested reader to other sources, for example, Bainbridge Cohen 2008, 2018; Stokes 2002; Hartley 1995.)

In essence, they are complex co-ordinations of alternating flexion and extension that support the infant to open out or gather in towards his centre. They are prerequisites for the full expression of the developmental movement patterns. They also underlie the fundamental impulses to *bond* – to move towards that which is desired and needed – or *defend* – to withdraw from or push away that which is not wanted or is feared; expressions of attraction and aversion are rooted in the primitive reflexes and responses.

One such reflex, the *Moro*, is present at birth. Also called the *startle reflex*, it is elicited by a shock; this could be a sudden change of position, a loud sound or bright light for example. Emergence at birth into a strange world of light and air and noise could certainly elicit a startle reflex.

In the first phase of the response the infant arches his spine, pulling his head back; his eyes and mouth open and he might cry. Arms are flung out to his sides, shoulders drawn in at the back, and legs might either extend or flex (depending on where they were before the startle).

If he is not safely gathered in and comforted, this pattern of extension, with contracted shoulders, head tipped back and mouth left open, might persist. This can leave an imprint for postural misalignment, tension in particular muscle groups and a tendency to be 'on alert', unable to calm and self-regulate after future shocks.

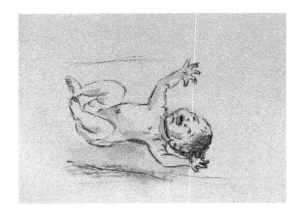
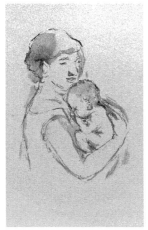

Figures 10.2 and 10.3: Moro Reflex – two phases. Artist: Raima Drąsutytė

After the first phase of the startle response, the infant needs to be supported and held so that he can release into the second phase: his arms open wide in order to flex into a full embrace; his neck flexes forward, allowing the mouth to close, and the whole body yields and relaxes into the reassuring embrace. Completion of the second phase of the Moro sets a template for a balanced autonomic nervous system where stress is balanced by safe holding, calming and comfort – sympathetic arousal is modulated by parasympathetic activation and social engagement, and a healthy cycle within the autonomic nervous system is restored.

Self and Other

I had been invited to lead a workshop at the Body-Mind Centering Association Conference, 2020, and was exploring connection to self and other as a core theme of my presentation. The process of gathering attention within and then opening out to the world is supported through the first months after birth by the integration of two responses: the *hand-to-mouth response* and the *asymmetric tonic neck reflex*. I decided to begin here.

Hand-to-mouth response:

I enter the process by lying on my back, allowing gravity to take my weight and my attention to be drawn into connection with the Earth. I yield and settle here for a while.

As I had been taught, many years before, I let my tongue gently reach to one side, inside my mouth, or simply follow the subtle falling of weight; I allow my head to turn towards that direction, then rest with my head on one side for a moment. I repeat this a few times from one side to the other, feeling how my whole body begins to curve in on the side I am turned towards, my spine laterally flexing and arms and legs following until the whole side rests in a flexed position. I keep my back body surface close to the floor as I turn my head, not rolling or twisting too much.

With each turn, my hand moves closer to my face, fingers and thumb naturally gravitating towards my mouth. My attention is drawn inside and I close my eyes. This is a familiar gesture for a young infant, offering a place of rest and turning of attention and sensing inwards. The infant can digest both food and experiences in this restful place. Many adults find this a comfortable position for sleep too.

Turning from one side to the other, the opposite side of my body naturally extends and opens; the hand rests on the floor above my head, my arm and leg lengthened away from centre. It becomes a whole-body movement, initiated by turning my head to one side then the other. My nervous system recognises this pattern, flexed along one whole side and extended along the other, and there is deep pleasure in the ease and familiarity of it. I continue for as long as feels right, turning side to side and deepening the sense of curling into myself.

In this moment I remember the first time I discovered the ease and fluidity of this movement pattern, during my Body-Mind Centering training over forty years ago. Then, as now, there was a sense that I could keep doing this forever, so natural and satisfying did it feel. I can still recall the studio, the exact place where I was lying on the floor, my practice partner sitting by my side, the feeling in my body just the same.

Asymmetric tonic neck reflex:

At some point I feel the moment of transition as the impulse to open out becomes strong. My eyes want to open and look out into the space around me. I turn and also extend my head back a little so that I am now looking out over my outstretched hand, arm extended above me along the floor. I have now turned towards the extended side; my vision guides the turning as I alternate from side to side, finding the whole-body pattern again.

I roll onto my belly and continue to explore the asymmetric tonic neck reflex, now feeling how the flexed side engages with the floor, ready to initiate a push from foot or hand. I feel more alert, present to what I am seeing in the space around me.

I continue to turn my head until I am back in the hand-to-mouth flexion pattern on the other side, then repeat to the first side. Turning from side to side, I feel the transition from the inward, restful focus of the hand-to-mouth, into a more active and externally engaged focus as my eyes are drawn to look out over my extended hand. The whole length of my body extends, from fingers to toes, while the opposite side naturally flexes in.

Once I fall into the rhythm of this alternation it feels so deeply nourishing, easeful and eventually graceful, that again I feel I could keep repeating this movement forever! I feel very at home here, my whole body connected and the balance between opening out to the world and returning inwards to self in finely tuned balance.

After a while the impulse to look out over my extended hand becomes stronger and I begin to crawl across the floor. The organic impulse to begin crawling, rolling and exploring the space, alternating with moments of rest, invites me into improvised movement.

The integration of these two responses gives underlying support to the balancing of the autonomic nervous system; it also enables the homolateral crawling pattern to emerge, and the infant's world expands as they can now move with agency and power towards what they desire.

Following this initial exploration, the intention of the workshop was to lead participants into embodied face-to-face movement explorations around sensing and feeling into boundaries and relationship through non-verbal channels. The initial practice was to serve as a preparation and resource for the exploration of the dynamic relationship between self and other. Sadly the covid pandemic led to the conference being cancelled, so this particular workshop never saw the light of day, but if you can follow my description above do try these movements for yourself and see what support they might give you.

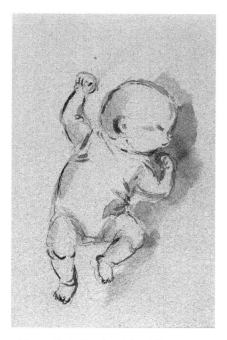

Figure 10.4: Hand-to-Mouth Response. Artist: Raima Drąsutytė

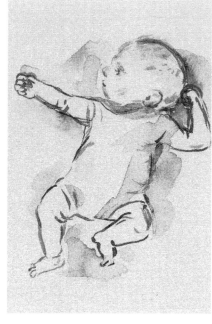

Figure 10.5: Asymmetric Tonic Neck Reflex. Artist: Raima Drąsutytė

To Summarise

The dynamic balance between opening out to the world and gathering back in towards self is one which we engage with from the very first moment of conception, and this challenge will be with us throughout life. Early development of the body's cells and tissues, its physiology, neurological processing and movement patterning involves increasingly complex ways in which we learn to navigate this dynamic relationship between self and other. Imprints are laid down and foundations embedded within our cells and tissues that will support, or hinder, our capacity to develop healthy relationships with others, and ultimately with Spirit too. Somatic practice can help us to become aware of and re-pattern unhelpful imprints or clarify and strengthen those imprints that resource us.

The sense of what constitutes 'other' is also evolving in complexity. At first the fluid matrix within the cell is in relation to the fluid matrix outside of the cell; they are distinct but not separate, fluid exchanging through a semi-permeable membrane, passing between the interior of the cell and the ocean that surrounds it. Here we begin to learn, experientially, about our intimate interweaving with and non-separation from the world around us. Our embodied being knows this as a reality.

Once the pre-embryo implants and begins to grow, 'other' becomes the mother's body, though it might not be felt to be separate. Gradually the little one will learn to differentiate herself from mother, first physically at birth, then psychologically as she develops. The world of 'other' becomes more complex, varied and vast as she grows. As the examples above describe, movement and physical development embody the essence of this journey of learning and engagement. They offer foundations for the experience of connecting to self and connecting to other, coming into relationship with the increasingly complex expressions of life that she will meet with throughout her journey. Ultimately relationship with Spirit may become known, and the duality of self and other may at times dissolve into *unitive consciousness*.

Part 4

Communication and Connectivity

11: Cellular Body

Having delved into how the individual human is formed and develops, and how boundaries of a sense of self emerge and are maintained throughout life, let us now look a little deeper at the ways in which those same boundaries might at times be expanded, transformed or dissolved, in both our perception of them and our embodied experience, allowing for fuller and more intimate connection with others, with the world we are a part of, and with Spirit.

Imagine a small pocket of ocean, a location both like and unlike every other part of the vast watery world that was home to the first cellular forms of life on Earth. It is thought that the first single-celled organisms evolved over 3.8 billion years ago, when swarms of congregating molecular processes formed around themselves a two-layered *phospholipid membrane*. Over aeons of time, functioning *organelles* evolved within the cell membrane; organelles 'breathe' and produce energy, proteins, enzymes, hormones and other essential substances, just as the organs of the body do on a larger scale. At all levels of existence, we see macrocosms reflected in microcosmic life: "[T]here is not one "new" function in our bodies that is not already expressed in the single cell" (Lipton 2008: 7). Included in these gatherings of microscopic structures were *mitochondria* and *chloroplasts*, which led to the special life forms of animal and plant respectively. They are thought to have evolved from bacteria: within our very cells live trillions of tiny structures of bacterial origin which power our every activity as they metabolise the energy we need to actively engage in life (Cooper 2000). They have their own DNA, which has the circular form of bacterial DNA rather than the human spirallic form (Barrett 2013: 108).

This discovery has challenged our sense of who we are. If our very capacity to be living beings with agency is because these 'others' are an integral part of us, of every cell in our bodies, then where do the boundaries of self *really* lie? We now know that the human body hosts vast colonies of bacterial microorganisms that contribute to our health and wellbeing in myriad ways, most significantly in the digestion of food; maintaining a healthy gut microbiome

(Ursell et al 2013) is a foundation of health in both body and mind. And, of course, at times invasion of harmful bacteria, viruses, fungi and other pathogens can overcome our defences and cause illness too, but these are usually temporary occurrences if treated appropriately. The bacteria which support life are an integral part of us; we cannot live without them and they cannot live without inhabiting our cells – the relationship is of mutually beneficial symbiosis.

We are connected to other life forms in more intimate ways than we could have previously imagined, and perhaps we are just beginning to feel comfortable with this reality as the notion of *Interbeing* settles more deeply in our collective mind. Whilst at a cellular level we can connect to the sense of being a contained and boundaried self (Juhan 1987: 21-2), and psychologically we need to develop this sense early in life, at the sub-cellular and molecular level we are far from that. Here we are 'many-as-one', an organismic template for the state of unitive consciousness perhaps, where boundaries between self and other fall away. Each cell is a community, just as each collection of cells that form a human body are a community; as in human society each cell, and each organelle within a cell, is playing its unique and crucial part in the symphony that is life.

As cell membranes formed around accumulations of molecular processes, enabling the organelles that power organic life to develop, communication between all that is contained within and all that lies outside became both possible and essential for life to unfold and evolve. The cell membrane acts as a place of transition and communication – sensitive, responsive, intelligent – the 'brain' of the cell, deciding what to welcome in and what to let go of (Lipton 2008: 45). As multi-celled organisms evolved, this capacity of the cellular membranes to listen and respond to each other's messages and needs became crucial for the co-ordinated functioning, health and development of the whole. This is as true for the first multi-cellular organisms and for the embryo in formation as it is for us as adult human beings.

The first methods of communication within the body are chemical processes, facilitated through the medium of inter- and intra-cellular fluids via intelligent cell membranes. As species evolved, and as we as individuals grew in complexity from our early embryonic days, this basic flow of molecular communication within the body continued to form the foundation of connectivity and organisation. Then, layered upon the flows of simpler chemical communication and response, in both species and embryo, more specific and focused systems evolved; they involved the production and release of molecules such as hormones and neuropeptides by particular cells. These are received by other specific cells, either throughout the whole body or at particular locations, which respond to them in very specific ways. This more sophisticated approach allowed great diversity, complexity and competence to flourish throughout the body.

The nervous system is the third layer of communication methods to evolve and develop. Faster, more specific and targeted, it integrates the slower processes of fluid-mediated molecular and hormonal messaging with lightning-quick electrical impulses. As Rupert Lipton describes, the organising and co-ordinating functions of the cellular 'mem-Brain' became the domain of the nervous system as species evolved. He notes: "It is not a coincidence that the human nervous system is derived from the embryonic skin, the human counterpart of a cell's membrane" (Lipton 2008: 58).

Whispering Between Cells

At the most fundamental level, communication within the body happens through the membranes of every cell. As cells breathe, taking in fluid, micronutrients and oxygen, and releasing wastes and chemical messengers, they subtly expand as the volume of fluid within their cytoplasmic body increases, and condense as fluid is released. This sets up a very subtle pulse, discernible through the microscope. This motility of the cells sends ripples out into the surrounding inter-cellular fluid, the internal ocean in which cells live. Imagine a group of thousands of cells pulsing in this way, their ripples bumping up against those of their neighbours, joining together and sending larger waves further out through the internal ocean. If the cells are at odds with each other this motion might be restless, chaotic, even turbulent. But cells that are coherently pulsing in rhythm with their neighbours send out a message of calm and cohesive stability. Healing and meditation practices seek to bring about such states of cellular coherence, often through *entraining* other bodily rhythms to pulse in harmony with each other – heart, external breathing, cerebrospinal rhythms, brain waves (Oschman 2000: 239). When cells are at ease within themselves and with each other they function with greater health and efficiency. The bodymind becomes more balanced and at ease, and can move towards greater health and wellbeing.

A simple exercise to entrain the rhythms of heart and breathing

- Kneeling or sitting comfortably – on a chair or cross-legged on a cushion – with your spine easily upright and free to move a little, take a few moments to settle your weight and begin to focus on your breathing. Feel its movement and rhythm.

- Internally count up to two, three, four, or whatever number is comfortable, as you breathe in; allow your spine to lengthen upwards.

- As you breathe out, again count to two, three or four; allow your spine to curve forwards, just as far as is comfortable.

- Continue for a few breaths like this. You might find the counting extends as your breathing deepens and slows.

- Can you sense the pulse of your heart beat beneath your breathing? Allow your counting to fall into this rhythm – approximately one beat per second. Lengthen up along your spine as you breathe in for four to six counts. Fold forwards as you breathe out for six to eight counts.

- Gradually the rhythms of your breathing and heart cohere so that it feels easy and natural to let them synchronise. This offers an invitation to all the cells of the body to cohere their pulse with the rhythms of heart and breath.

Cells also communicate with each other through the chemical signals they send out into the wider fluid environment. As noted above, some cells are designed to produce specific chemicals such as hormones, which stimulate certain other cells to change their behaviour – perhaps to produce their own chemical messengers, such as enzymes, hormones or neuropeptides, or to become more or less active. A multi-directional whispered conversation is taking place amongst the cells of the whole body, an endless conversation that regulates all of our physiological and also emotional and psychological processes.

When Candace Pert's book *Molecules of Emotion* was first published in 1997, she opened the world of scientific research into molecular messaging to a wider audience of lay and professional readers. Practitioners in the healing and therapeutic communities eagerly embraced her work as it brought deepened awareness and scientific validation to the intuited sense of interconnectedness between body, emotions, thought and imagination that they were working with. Beyond this, she also recounted the story of one woman's struggles in a male-dominated scientific environment and, more than that – a female scientist who believed that the secrets of life, health and illness could only be unravelled through inter-disciplinary research. The old way (traditionally the way of male-dominated patriarchal structures and thinking) of studying aspects of human biology and behaviour in compartmentalised boxes of knowledge could only take us so far. Pert was one of the pioneers who broke open those boxes and looked into the inter-relationships between the nervous, immune and endocrine systems, mind, emotions and their integrative impact on illness and health. I am sure it is no coincidence that a woman played such a central role in this upturning of the old paradigm to usher in new ways of approaching the lived experience of body and mind that held relatedness and connectivity at their heart.

In the study of Body-Mind Centering we first learn to differentiate each body system, embodying its specific and unique qualities of expression and support. This is a valuable step in getting to know our less familiar 'shadow' systems, bringing them into expression and re-balancing the way we organise our soma and psyche (Bainbridge Cohen 1993; Hartley 1995, 2004). But, of course, they do not work in isolation. It is in the integration of the systems that psyche-soma truly comes alive. The work of Pert and her colleagues, in the interface between disciplines and physiological systems, has supported a deeper understanding of the relationship between our body's chemistry, physiology and the emotions that surge through us.

Her research into *neuropeptides* revealed fascinating information and contributed to a paradigmatic shift in how we think about psyche and soma, mind and body. Neuropeptide molecules that are produced in the brain and received by other brain cells affect mood and feeling states; they also travel around the body. She and her colleagues discovered that there are neuropeptide receptor sites on the cell membranes of immune and endocrine cells throughout the body, as well as those of brain cells; neuropeptides link the brain, immune and endocrine systems through the flow of information between them. And furthermore, neuropeptides are also produced, stored and secreted by immune cells throughout the body: mood altering chemical messengers flow from immune cells to the brain, as well as from the brain to immune and other cells (Pert 1997: 182-3). Her research led her to the view that:

> [M]ind is the flow of information as it moves among the cells, organs, and systems of the body ... The mind as we experience it is immaterial, yet it has a physical substrate, which is both the body and the brain. It may also be said to have a nonmaterial, nonphysical substrate that has to do with the flow of that information. The mind, then, is that which holds the network together. (Pert 1997: 185)

Here is another experiment you might like to try. In exploring the embodiment of immune cells and their potential to alter mood, I imagined being one single immune cell travelling through the blood circulation, as they do for some or all of their life. What I felt was a great surge of joy and fun as I 'became' the cell, bursting out of the contained space of the ventricles of the heart into the aorta, diving up and over through the aortic arch, then swooshing down and through the body. Sometimes slow and calm, pausing to rest for a moment in the *capillary isorings* where exchange between blood and cells takes place (Hartley 1995: 275), at other times rushing and racing headlong, the journey of a single cell through the network of blood vessels is truly a marvellous one, with many twists, turns and, when embodied as I describe below, the potential to elicit emotional highs and lows. It might even feel as if the cell itself is 'happy or joyful, sad or anxious' as it journeys through the body. We can imagine this to be the case if we understand the cell to possess its own awareness, and to be a microcosm of the body as a whole; embodying, becoming one with the cell as Bonnie Bainbridge Cohen describes, we can experience the journey through the blood stream with the cell.

An experiment in embodying an immune cell

- ➤ Focus your attention towards your blood circulation. Go inside the vessels. Choose one place to begin and 'enter into' the presence of a single white blood cell. This is done first through your imagination, but if you can engage with this fully you may begin to sense and feel a deeper embodiment taking place.

- ➤ Let yourself be carried – through the chambers of the heart where there is a moment of rest; pumped through the vessels that reach out to the lungs, circulating the narrow and delicate passageways that encircle the alveoli sacs within the lungs, looking out for infectious pathogens; back into the heart, held in stillness for a moment; then propelled with some force out of the heart again, up and over the aortic arch. Following the 1-2 rhythmic beat of the heart, blood flows at about sixty miles per hour when it first leaves the heart, gradually slowing down as it travels to the furthest reaches of the cellular body. Enjoy the ride! See where it takes you, into which nook and cranny of the body.

- ➢ Continue the return journey, blood moving more slowly to the 1-2-3 rhythm of a waltz, back to the heart where the cycle begins again.

- ➢ Allow the feelings of the journey to move you – let the dance of the immune cell within you be amplified into a dance of your whole body.

If immune cells, when embodied in such ways as this, are experienced as 'happy' this might affect our whole mood in a positive way. And feelings of happiness, we know, can support the immune system. Benign and healing cycles of mutual enhancement between brain, psyche, immune system and endocrine system can be established. Conversely, stress, anger, fear and other strong emotions can adversely affect our immunity if they are held onto for too long and not resolved.

The Emotional Brain and Psycho-neuro-immuno-endocrinology

The effects of the mind and emotions on the health and sickness of the body has been a subject of exploration for millennia, from the shamanic practices of indigenous cultures, to the sacred healing rituals of the ancient Greeks, and more recently the explorations of psychiatry, psychoanalysis and the many branches of psychotherapy and therapeutic hypnosis that have evolved from them. Thought, emotion and imagination profoundly influence physiological function and expression. Like Pert, Ernest Lawrence Rossi was researching in the interstices between disciplines as the field of psychoneuroimmunology (PNI) was evolving. He saw that mind and the various 'messenger' systems of the body are intimately connected, and his book *The Psychobiology of Mind-Body Healing* seeks to trace the astonishingly complex co-ordinations that are constantly taking place between them. He believes that the endocrine system should really be included in the naming of psychoneuroimmunology, as it is an essential part of the interweaving pathways of information processing.

His research led him to consider the question of a mind-gene connection: the effect of mind not only on observable physiological processes and emotional expression, but on the very nature of the genes and molecules within the cells. As one example, he writes:

> Under "mental" stress, the limbic-hypothalamic system in the brain converts the neural messages of mind into the neurohormonal "messenger molecules" of the body. These, in turn, can direct the endocrine system to produce steroid hormones that can reach into the nucleus of different cells of the body to modulate the expression of genes. These genes then direct the cells to produce the various molecules that will regulate metabolism, growth, activity level, sexuality, and the immune response in sickness and health ... Mind ultimately does modulate the creation and expression of the molecules of life! (Rossi 1986: xiv)

He describes in some detail how mind modulates the autonomic nervous, endocrine, immune and neuropeptide systems of the body, opening pathways towards health and balance. In the decades since Rossi's work was published, the fields of affective neuroscience and psychoneuroimmunology have gathered breathtaking amounts of information about the connectivity between mind, emotion and the body. The work of brilliant researchers and writers such as Allan Schore (1994), Antonio Damasio (1994) and Joseph LeDoux (1998) have greatly contributed to our understanding of brain function and emotion, and the development of psychosocial relationships. New paradigms have evolved which place emotional and relational interaction at the heart of healing processes.

Meanwhile, the field of somatics has been exploring the other side of this dance – how body affects mind: the effects of touch and movement upon our emotions, thoughts and imagination, and also our access to spiritual experiences. Our whole body, from skin surface to the nuclear heart of every cell, is like a complex antenna, constantly picking up, attuning and responding to the calls of the environment. This information affects mind, emotion, memory and imagination in both harmful and healing ways. We are not conscious of most of the information that is reaching us, or the impact it is having upon us, but somatic practice can train us to develop conscious awareness of the messages from our environment, both human and non-human, so as to better support benign and healing cycles.

Research into digestive processing within the human gut also supports the *body-mind* direction of the flow of information. In *The Second Brain* Michael Gershon (1998) describes the discovery of the *enteric nervous system*, which functions independently of the brain of the central nervous system. He writes about the discovery of the presence of an extensive and highly complex network of nerve cells that co-ordinate digestive activity, independently of the brain, though in communication with it. The enteric nervous system uses primary cellular-fluid and reflexive processing; it also interacts with the endocrine system and autonomic nervous system, which creates direct links between gut health and mental health. If our gut is functioning well this will be reflected in our mental and emotional states too.

Energetic Pathways

In his wide-reaching research into *Energy Medicine* (2000) James Oschman describes other subtle ways in which communication within the body, between cells and tissues, occurs. I first encountered Oschman's work at a Zero-Balancing conference in London (June 2000), where I and other bodywork therapists were intrigued and inspired by his accounts of research that offered ways of validating the practices of healing through touch. One aspect of our internal communication network is the all-pervasive system of connective tissue; in its various forms it envelops, differentiates and penetrates every tissue of the body. It wraps around the whole body as the sub-cutaneous fascial layer, and travels deep inside around muscles, bones, nerves, blood and lymph vessels, organs and glands; it connects bone and muscle as ligament and tendon; it circulates as fluid connective tissue in the form of interstitial fluid, blood and lymph, and more. Microfilaments of connective tissue also surround and enter the very cells, forming a 'living matrix': intra-cellular networks of micro fibres provide the supportive internal *cytoskeleton* of the cell, and facilitate the passage of essential molecules between cell membrane, organelles and nucleus (see *Figure 8:1*).

Micro fibres also enter the nucleus itself, surrounding the genetic material that is housed there (Oschman 2000: 46). "In essence, when you touch a human body, you are touching a continuously interconnected system, composed of virtually all of the molecules in the body linked together in an intricate webwork" (Oschman 2000: 48). Connective tissue is an efficient conductor of magnetic and electrical energy, so when the skin is touched information can reach deep into the heart and brain of every cell. The quality of attention and intention that the touch holds communicates directly with the heart of the cells being contacted. When the touch of a healer or body therapist focuses towards specific groups of cells an energetic resonance is established between their hands and the tissue being contacted. The cells respond positively to touch that expresses love, compassion, care and the intention to support healing (Oschman 2000: 91).

Oschman suggests that Pert's detailed work on the chemical messaging of neuropeptides can be integrated with studies into electromagnetic flow and resonance within the body. Electrical charges pass through the living matrix virtually instantaneously, opening up new possibilities for understanding cellular and tissue communication and healing. We probably have much still to discover about communication and interaction within humans and between humans and other organisms at a quantum level. Oschman writes:

> *In the past we thought the words of the 'language of life' were nerve impulses and molecules, but we now see that there is a deeper layer of communication underlying these familiar processes. Beneath the relatively slow-moving action potentials and billiard ball interactions of molecules lies a much faster and subtle realm of interactions. This dimension is subatomic, energetic, electromagnetic and wave-like in character. The chemical messenger ultimately transfers its information electromagnetically.*
> (Oschman 2000: 251)

This virtually instantaneous way of communicating results in *resonance*, the simultaneous occurrence of vibration within tissues at different locations in the body (or between bodies). One pathway of resonance which I have found particularly fascinating and powerful is that which occurs between the double helix structure of DNA within the heart of each cell, and the similar double-helix formation of the single band of muscle that forms the heart[1]. When consciousness is brought to them, they might be felt to mutually vibrate, the way the string of a violin and a tuning fork do when perfectly tuned. If you like, you can try this experiment:

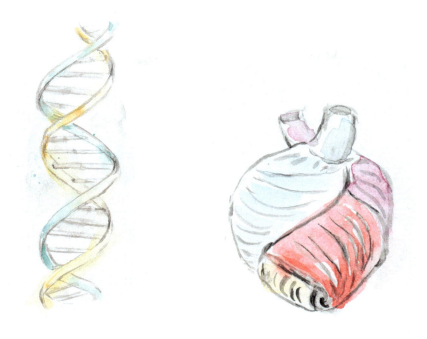

Figures 11.1: DNA and Heart Muscle as a Double Helix. Artist: Raima Drąsutytė

Meditation for heart and DNA

➢ Find a comfortable place to sit or lie down and take a few moments to ground, relax, breathe and open to the presence of the internal respiration of your cells.

➢ Place one hand gently over your heart to support awareness there. Place your other hand on an area of your body that is calling for attention – perhaps a place that holds tension or pain. If it is not possible or comfortable to place your hand there, then simply hold that place in your awareness.

➢ Let the cells in both locations breathe as fully as they can in this moment, opening to their own presence within the body.

> Now visualise the double-helix form of the heart muscle, spiralling around itself in a continuous loop. Then include in your awareness the same double-helix structure of the spiralling DNA within the nuclei of the cells beneath your other hand (or held in your awareness).

> Rest in this dual awareness of the heart spiral and the spiral of DNA within the cells.

When I first tried this simple experiment, I was astonished at its effect. I felt an immense expansion of consciousness, boundaries falling away to allow an experience of inner and outer becoming one, my mind opening to a spaciousness that felt profound and healing. It is different every time; your own experience will be different too. Allow it to be whatever it is.

The Cell's Code of Three

Sondra Barrett expands the idea of resonance to embrace and link together the cell's genetic code, the three embryological germ layers, and the symbols and myths of religions and cultures around the world. She describes how the DNA 'code of three' is at the root of the creation of life: to build the proteins which are the foundation of cellular birth, growth and repair, amino acids are formed; this requires that three out of the four basic molecules that form our DNA come together. The 'code of three' is also active in genetic expression and in the creation of the cell's structure where multiples of three are found: "[C]ellular creation requires a 3^3 tube-like structure (centriole) to guide the way" (Barrett 2013: 184). The *trinity* also appears in embryological development as the three germinal layers form, out of which all subsequent structures will evolve; and of course the womb container is a three-layered membrane, as we have seen. The *triune brain* evolves too, (though it should be noted that brain function is far more complex than this theory suggests[2]): "The reptilian brain stem provides for essential survival mechanisms; the limbic system gives us our emotional, nurturing capabilities; and the most recent addition, the outer cortex, enables us to think and reason" (Barrett 2013: 185).

Widening out her perspective, she suggests connection and resonance within the symbology of many of the world's cultures and religions – Christianity's *Trinity*, Judaism's *Three faces of God*, ancient Greece's *Gaia, Eros and Thanatos*, the *Triple Jewel* of *Buddha, Dharma and Sangha* in

Buddhism, and many more. In archetypal psychology we find the trinity of *Maiden, Mother and Crone,* and the *transcendent function,* the third position that integrates two polarities to bring us to a place of greater integration and higher evolution. We find this integration within the dance of polarities as the embryo forms: first, the sperm and egg come together to make the *zygote*, mother and father to make a child. Here integration itself *is* the third pole, which creates balance, new life and evolution. The triangle is also found in abundance in sacred geometry, suggesting the centrality of *three-fold* in the subtle structuring of reality.

The cell's 'code of three', the foundational principle for the generation of life in all its forms, seems to inspire and be reflected in all levels of embodied and mystical creation. Or we could put this the other way – the mysticism of the law of three is present within the very origins of cellular life, linking diverse expressions of life in mysterious ways.

12: Earth Body

Earth moves, spinning through space in her daily and seasonal cycles – a dance with sun, moon, stars and the space she revolves within, renewing and recycling every form of life that inhabits her through these infinitely repeating motions.

Scientists tell us that long ago – maybe 335 million years ago – Earth consisted of one solid land mass amidst the enveloping ocean[1]. They called this ancient body Pangaea. I like to imagine the transformation of Pangaea into Earth as we know her today as a movement of breath. Pangaea breathed in. She filled and rose up, plates shifted apart and the continents were formed. Perhaps one day Earth will complete her out breath, land will settle and there will be one single land mass again.

Earth breathes. Earth is alive. We can come to know Earth, Gaia, as a conscious living being, and even imagine that she, like us, is awakening to conscious embodied movement as she sends storms, floods, fires, earthquakes and volcanoes, even tiny viruses, as messages to us to pay attention. To listen deeply. To heed the warnings.

James Lovelock first introduced the modern world to the concept of Gaia as a living system, and in the decades since the publication of *Gaia* (Lovelock 1991) a wealth of scientific information about the deep interconnectedness of planetary ecosystems has emerged. We are learning more and more about the interactions between soil, trees, climate, ice caps and sea, animals, insects, fish and birds, and humans; we are discovering how these interactions support a healthy ecology, enabling great diversity of plant and animal species to flourish, when Nature is allowed to take her own course. At the same time, we have been discovering how cells, tissues and systems within the body interact as one inseparable whole, forming a deep ecology of interconnectedness within that reflects the "wood wide web" (Sheldrake 2020: 190) that we are part of.

Indigenous cultures have always perceived and lived in close relationship with the intelligent systems which govern all life on Earth, including human life. For them, Nature in all its forms is alive, intelligent and worthy of our respect and deep care. We modern humans have largely lost the sense of respect and reverence towards Nature which is so central to the worldview and practices of indigenous peoples, but as the current climate and ecological crisis impinges more urgently upon our consciousness, we are being called to re-engage with the perennial wisdom of our ancestors and those who still follow the path of treading gently on sacred Earth.

> *Science is evolving, recognizing that nature is composed of interdependent systems within systems within systems, just as a human body is; that soil mycorrhizal networks are as complex as brain tissue; that water can carry information and structure; that the earth and even the sun maintain homeostatic balance just as a body does. We are learning that order, complexity, and organization are fundamental properties of matter, mediated through physical processes that we recognize – and perhaps by others we do not. The excluded spirit is coming back to matter, not from without but from within.* (Eisenstein 2018: 258)

Whispering Between Trees

Just as Pert, Oschman and other researchers have been revealing the mysteries of connectedness and integration within the body and between body and mind, physiological body systems, and the movement of energy and the flow of intelligence within the human being, others have been delving into the connections between plants, fungi, bacteria and the communications that go on, invisible to our human gaze, across the natural world. Networks as complex and mysterious as those within an individual organism are to be found everywhere around us.

Merlin Sheldrake's title *Entangled Lives* (2020) imaginatively evokes the complex and miraculous network that is Nature. He describes the critical role that fungi play in connecting life forms and enabling growth. There is an intimate attraction between tree roots and fungi; fungal hyphae branch throughout the roots, forming a mycorrhizal network deep beneath the forest floor that connects individual trees and plants into a community. The mycorrhizal network is vast, pervasive and intricate, forming pathways through which communication, nourishment, water and healing can flow amongst trees and plants. Bacteria are also involved in these processes which fungi enable. "Mycelium is ecological connective tissue, the living seam by which much of the world is stitched into relation" (Sheldrake 2020: 52). It is movement which enables these connections, the tips of fungal hyphae travelling through soil, growing around and along tree roots, rocks, branches.

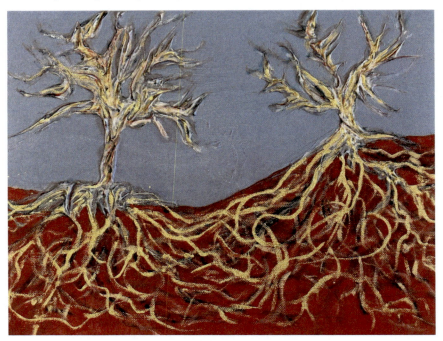

Figure 12:1. 'Roots'. Artist: Brue Richardson

In *Finding the Mother Tree* (2021) ecologist Suzanne Simard describes trees as social beings. Just like human beings and other non-human animals, they are designed to relate to each other within living communities and, as she describes, they are nourished by a central 'mother tree' at the heart of the community, an old and established tree which directs support and resources to less resilient young saplings.

> *A linchpin in the tree-fungi networks are hub trees. Also referred to as "mother trees," these are the older, more seasoned trees in a forest. Typically, they have the most fungal connections. Their roots are established in deeper soil, and can reach deeper sources of water to pass on to younger saplings. Through the mycorrhizal network, these hub trees detect the ill health of their neighbors from distress signals, and send them needed nutrients.* (Holewinski: online)

The intelligence of this is remarkable. We are not unique; trees, plants and fungi form communities just as animals – from ants, to wolves, to wild geese, to humans – do. As the psychology of attachment theory and Porges' *social engagement system* have shown us, we are interdependent, helped and nourished by our social interactions with each other, and so are the trees.

When we speak of intelligence, we generally speak from our human perspective, equating intelligence with the specific form of cognitive processing which the human brain and central nervous system support. We use this bar when we assess the intelligence of other mammals too – how close is their intelligence to ours? But we are learning that we must expand our ideas of intelligence if we are to understand the world we inhabit more fully, and be able to act in ways that will help to sustain its health. One definition of intelligence is "the ability to learn or understand or to deal with new or trying situations"[2]. This surely encompasses the complex ways in which Nature's eco-systems function and thrive – the discerning activity of cellular membranes, the co-habitation and support networks of fungi and trees, the art of pollination which bees and other insects excel in, the migratory patterns of birds, and so on. The deep intelligence of the human and non-human organism, of Nature in her myriad interdependent life forms and of Gaia as a living ecosystem whose intelligent functioning is still way beyond our full comprehension – all of this asks of us humility and respect.

We are Earth

> *Besides sharing the same DNA coding system with all other living creatures and plants, we all use the same elemental chemicals of carbon, hydrogen, oxygen, nitrogen, sulfur, and phosphorus as the basis of life ... We are joined together by sharing the same elusive quantum physics, molecular DNA, and the essence of cellular life.*
> (Barrett 2013: 194)

We humans are completely embedded in the *web of life*. We are of the Earth, made of the same elements, not separate but an integral part. In our bones are the minerals that form the bedrock of the Earth. Blood also contains iron, which is drawn towards the magnetic core of the Earth, drawing us to her. Our bodily fluids originate from the same ocean that envelops Earth – cellular and interstitial fluids are the medium within which life can flourish, amniotic fluid supports the growing embryo and foetus, lymph helps protect us from injury and disease, cerebrospinal fluid bathes and nourishes our nervous system. Organic life takes place within the shared medium of the ocean of the world. We breathe in oxygen which trees and plants exhale, giving us the energetic fire that fuels life; and we exhale carbon dioxide which sustains the plants – what a miracle of interdependence is this! We humans are an intimately interdependent part of the living network of processes which is Gaia.

Our matter is inseparable from the matter of Earth. We, like other animate creatures, are expressions of Earth with the ability to move about on her surface, to leap and fly above her for a while, or bury beneath her surface. I think of us as an aspect of Earth body with the capacity to express freely through movement. We are Earth dancing – a different quality of dance from the trees who are swayed gracefully by the wind whilst staying, steadfast, patient, rooted to one place throughout their lives – our dance no more or less beautiful. And perhaps through this dance Earth is becoming conscious through us.

But what of our consciousness, our Spirit, our embodied awareness? It is here that we humans can feel ourselves to be different, separate. We think, we analyse and imagine, we feel emotion, exercise will and agency, but we have to a considerable extent lost touch with the innate intelligence of Nature that binds all living systems together; we have developed capacities to override some of the natural cycles of Earth's ecosystems to suit our own human ambitions, at great cost. Knowing that our future and the health of our home the Earth depend on recovering our connectivity with Nature, some look to the wisdom of indigenous cultures, to natural healing practices, organic and regenerative farming, the philosophy of compassion and *Interbeing* which Buddhism and other religions cultivate. And what can somatic practices contribute to this movement to heal our connection with our environment? What has the practice of conscious embodiment to offer?

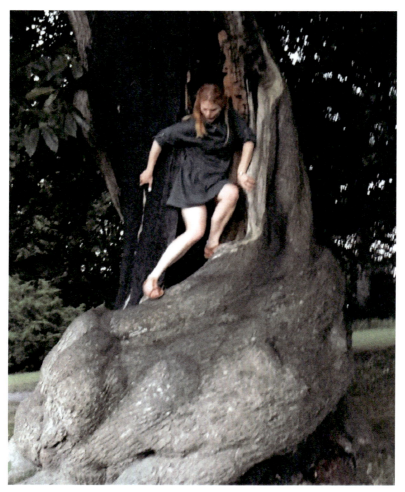

Figure 12.2: Barbara Erber, participant in IBMT Gathering at Dartington Hall, Devon, July 2018. Photo: Linda Hartley

Whilst we feel separate from Earth and Nature, the respect and love of life that would impel us to treat all of its manifestations as equal to our own may not arise. Even in the current atmosphere of concern about climate change, ecosystem degradation, and the extinction of many species, the bottom line is so often 'how can Earth and Nature best serve our needs, how can we save the planet so that we can survive upon it?' – not 'how can we save all life on Earth purely for its own sake, because all beings deserve the same right to life as we do?'

When we come to feel, in a deep and embodied way, that we are an integral part of this miraculous phenomenon that is Gaia, these concerns can start to shift. Instead of the quest to save the planet so that we can survive, pure love of the raw beauty, majesty, intelligence and complexity of earthly life can begin to inform our thoughts and actions.

> *I am kneeling, the hollows of my palms circling around my knees, cupping the bones. My body is rocking slowly forwards and backwards with this movement.*
>
> *My hands come to rest. I feel the solidity of bone beneath my hands, the perfect fit of hollow palms cupping rounded bones. At first the bone feels cold, hard, 'not-me'. It is Earth. Bone is of the Earth, contains the minerals of the Earth, their hardness, their supportive structure. If I do not feel part of the Earth, then my bones are 'not-me'.*
>
> *I am searching for 'me' in my body.*
>
> *Now my wrists meet and are circling around each other, slowly, circling around the question, 'Where in my body am I?' In this moment I don't find 'me'. But I become conscious of wrist knowing wrist, bone knowing flesh, skin knowing joint.*
>
> *I know that bone contains cells, fluids and soft tissues too. I begin to connect with bone through these presences. Gradually I come to feel embodied as bone-as-living-tissue and this opens a path to experience bone in its wholeness – mineral, fluid, fibre, cell. I am connecting to the consciousness of bone in my body, and now I meet the consciousness of the bones of the Earth, the bedrock of minerals beneath me intertwined with the living matrix of soil, tree roots and fungi.*
>
> *I come to feel that Earth is conscious, and it is because of this that I can consciously embody my mineral bones. Because the waters, the air and the fire are conscious, I can consciously embody the fluids and tissues and fire within me, which originate in the elements of Nature that create my embodied self.*
>
> *My bones now feel soft, warm, supple, alive. I am present within them and equally I am present within the rock of the Earth, and Earth is present within me. We are no longer separate.*
>
> (Excerpt from my Authentic Movement journal)

When I deeply feel my connection, my embodied at-oneness with Earth and Nature, the sense of separateness can begin to transform towards feeling an integral part of. The *idea* of minerals and salty brine and oxygen within me being shared with all other life forms can settle down from being a mental concept to becoming an embodied, experienced reality. After the movement session described above, I am filled with a feeling of deep peace and wonder, a place where need and desire can rest and presence grow.

Somatic movement and Authentic Movement practice offer ways of coming into direct embodied connectivity with Earth and the natural world. This engenders in practitioners a genuine love, awe, respect and desire to care for Gaia.

More and more I hear students in my teaching practice speaking of *being*, rather than *feeling like* or *seeing an image of* some part of the natural world: not "I feel like a tree" but "I am a tree, with roots reaching deep into the Earth"; "I am an eagle soaring high above the land, seeing with an eagle's eye", rather than "I have an image of an eagle flying"; "I am a worm, I know how it is to be a worm burrowing into the Earth"; "I am rock".

In a recent retreat five women had gathered for several days to practise the Discipline of Authentic Movement in my studio. In one session, all five choose to be movers. From the very first moment, as the bell rings and they each close their eyes, I sense a deep quality of stillness, concentration and connection between all five of them. This continues without a break for the whole fifty minutes of moving time. I feel both alert and deeply absorbed as I witness. Throughout most of the time they are in physical contact, sometimes all five in a loosely connected circle, sometimes in a crescent with just a small opening. Light, tender touches of hands, feet, a head, sometimes the side of the ribs, not imposing or demanding, just a recognition of presence and connection. For most of the time four of the women move close to the floor, while the fifth stands tall amidst them. The quality of connectedness between them makes me think of the mycorrhizal network beneath the forest floor, those intricately woven threads of communication, nourishment and healing that the trees and plants engage in.

During the speaking and listening circle afterwards they confirm this sense of connection, each naming her part in the collective process while delving deep into her own experience. One mover describes her experience in this way:

I am kneeling with my hands on my lap, very still and hardly breathing. I am strong and committed.

I am a rock.

My anger is sealed deep inside, which becomes an epicentre of the condensing force.

I notice a bird stops by on my knee then my shoulder.

Someone's touch gently invites me to respond.

I hear the song of the wind.

Tones of voice and breath flow above me.

Someone is sliding on my right side and passing. A stream.

I become a willow tree just for now, then I return to being a rock.

I stay here hard and still while sensing and feeling all happening around me.

I may be the fulcrum.

Over time, I notice my stiff fingers softening and also my skin.

Now I know that I am alive.

My aliveness needs slow time.

Amongst all the birds, wind and stream, I am also changing.

Living.

This is how I participate in the world.

And now I know how a rock feels.

(Retreat participant Katsura Isobe – with permission)

Another writes in her journal and shares:

> *I am standing. My feet are planted on the floor, my face is reaching to the light. My right hand is cupped, honouring humility. My left-hand fingers meet at their tips. My hand is bud.*
>
> *Another mover's hand rests on my right foot. The present staying connection of this mover allows my feet, legs, to drop deep into the earth. Roots reach down.*
>
> *I am tree.*
>
> *Around me movers are rock. Movers are connected. Moss. Mycelium.*
>
> *Gentle breath sounds come from my mouth, wind through branches.*
>
> *My budded fingers slowly reach up and open towards the light, until my palm and fingers stretch wide in bloom.*
>
> *We are forest. The space opens around me.*
>
> (Retreat participant Rebecca Hastings – with permission)

Another mover describes her flowing movement becoming *stream* as she moves gently along the side of the *rock* and is tumbled towards the *tree*. The other two movers are close by, deeply engaged in delicate, tender touches as they explore their inner worlds whilst also holding the circle of movers strong.

Earth as Witness

I can locate my own awakening to the plight of Earth at the hands of humanity to one particular train journey early in 1987, as I travelled from the Buddhist retreat centre where I had been staying, back to my home in London. I remember the profound grief that was welling up in me, growing with each mile of the journey from green fields and woodlands to ever more urbanised landscapes. The grass seemed to become less green, more sparse. More grey industrial units and bland housing estates sprung up to replace it. Clean air was replaced by the impression of dirt and soot and the detritus of life carelessly thrown away, sticking to the grey walls of factories, shopping centres and impoverished neighbourhoods. It felt like a journey from paradise to purgatory. By the time I reached London my grief was complete, and my conviction that we humans had created this devastating loss of Nature filled me with despair. I had undoubtedly been struck in this way because I had been opened at this particular time to the full consciousness of my own hidden pain. In this raw place I was open to experiencing the pain of others in a more intimate way than ever before; a deepened empathic resonance with other people and with the suffering of the Earth and Nature had awakened.

Not long after this I experienced a truly conscious connection with Mother Earth as witness; it was during a period of deep pain and grief which grew out of my own life's losses as well as the welling up grief for Earth and Nature. I was back at the retreat centre in the countryside. I had gone into the garden to seek solace, unable at that moment to find human comfort. Lying on my belly on the grass, hidden by trees, I allowed myself to sob deeply into the Earth. Almost immediately I felt embraced by a profound wave of compassion, surrounding and washing through me. It was absolutely clear to me that this loving witness was the Earth herself. I felt totally and unconditionally accepted in a way that I had never experienced before. My relationship with conscious Earth began to grow from this time.

Robin Wall Kimmerer writes:

> *Knowing that you love the earth changes you, activates you to defend and protect and celebrate. But when you feel that the earth loves you in return, the feeling transforms the relationship from a one-way street into a sacred bond.* (Kimmerer 2013: 124)

At the heart of the Discipline of Authentic Movement is the cultivation of a loving, compassionate and accepting witness within. Essential to this process is the presence of another who has travelled the path before us, an external witness who can see us with enough clarity and compassion. Moving in her presence, over time we gradually internalise the loving and compassionate witness; a place of clear awareness within is sourced. Authentic Movement is a relational practice – through relationship with another we come into deepened relationship with ourself, and through this we in turn deepen and expand our sense of connection with others, with Nature, Earth and the Sacred in its many expressions.

During much of the time that I was working on this book, the lockdowns necessitated by the pandemic meant that many of us who practise Authentic Movement were unable to meet to practise together. For some, sessions by video link have substituted for the embodied presence of another in the studio. For others, solo practice has deepened.

My practice space is my garden studio. It overlooks a field and is loosely surrounded by trees – oak, willow, fir, rowan. The skylight windows look up into the sky and the branches of an oak tree grace this view. Birds visit for a while or fly swiftly by, and their song is an accompaniment to my movement. During this time of intensified solo practice my relationship with the Nature that surrounds the studio has grown.

I watched this studio space being created. First, a great deal of rubbish, some dead trees and shrubs, and three old garden sheds had to be cleared. It was tempting to leave the space that was revealed open and empty. The view over the fields invited settling into spaciousness and quiet – I could have left it just like this, a quiet, empty space to reflect in. But I continued with my dream of building the studio. Once the timber frame was up, again I was tempted to leave it as an open structure; I loved being in this open space, the wind blowing through and late afternoon sunlight filtering in through the upright wooden supports. Having known the building like this, I had such a clear sense of the walls, once they were installed, as being no more than a thin membrane containing some of the external space within them. From the beginning the boundary between the space within the studio and the vast space outside felt transparent, the separation barely present. Now, when I move in the studio, with its windows on three sides and above, and trees all around, I feel close to Nature.

My sense of Earth as witness deepened during this period of sustained time at home and solo practice. What I have come to experience as Earth's witness consciousness often expresses through the birds and trees, sometimes through clouds, rain, sun or wind. On a number of occasions I have opened my eyes at the end of a movement session, looking up through the skylight window to see a bird – wood pigeon, blackbird, robin – sitting on a branch of the oak tree, looking down at me. Head tilted slightly to one side, one eye looks directly at me. I cannot ascribe interest or curiosity – that would be to attempt to humanise a wild bird's experience – but it is clearly looking at me and seeing me. I feel met.

The oak tree behind the studio has a strong presence that often pulls me towards it. With eyes closed, I often find myself sitting or standing by the wall behind which Oak stands, perhaps leaning into the tree's support, or bowing to it. Occasionally kneeling and praying for help. We have gradually grown an intimate relationship. It has a quality that I could call 'masculine' – clear, direct, unsentimental but strong and supportive – though again, I am at risk of humanising the tree by ascribing human qualities. If I listen attentively, I may receive messages that offer guidance or comfort or inspiration.

Oak has been particularly present for me during this time. Jacqueline Memory Paterson describes how: "According to Nature mystics of all ages, the oak is a doorway … Through these doorways we enter other dimensions where we perceive different realities and worlds." (1996: 189) The magnificent Oak that stands at the edge of a neighbour's land, a small distance in front of my studio, I have come to know as Grandmother Oak. In my movement practice I often find myself facing her as I connect with the ancestors, my grandmothers. Teacher Oak began to call me strongly as the pandemic began and my daily walks were limited to the lane that led from my house to this tree. Later, pain in my body began to limit my walking capacity and I could no longer reach her; then following surgery she became a marker, the goal I set myself until gradually I could reach Teacher Oak again. A large spreading tree with solid upright trunk, I sensed her imposing presence as conveying a wordless message – her stillness, endurance and the broken branches that hung around her base taught me about enduring through the pain and brokenness in myself and in the world. Teacher Oak remained steadfast, unmoving and strong through all weathers and endless stretches of time, even as old and damaged branches died and fell from her. She was teaching me to embrace all of it.

Along the horizon, across the field at the front of the studio, stands a row of trees, also oak. I see three of these through the windows, clear shapes against the sky, their innermost branches covered in ivy that gives each a distinct and unusual shape. Sometimes they greet me, as I open my eyes at the end of a movement session, in such a way that I feel witnessed by them. One has a wide embrace of branches which brings me to, and reflects back to me, feelings of compassion and kindness; another has an energetic upward reach that I feel as inspiring and energising, and have felt my own movement and feelings mirrored by this uplifting gesture; the third has fine dancing 'fingers' emerging from boughs densely covered by a mass of ivy – they evoke a light and joyful feeling, they make me smile.

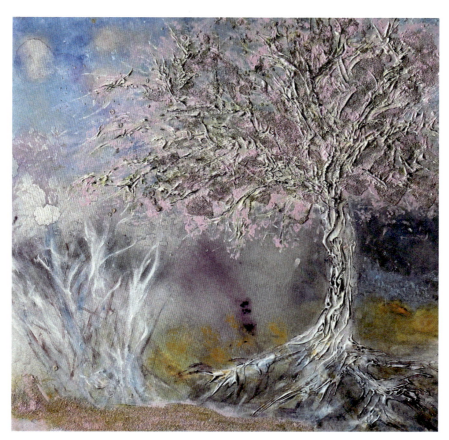

Figure 12.3: 'Spring'. Artist: Brue Richardson

Towards the end of the moving time, my hands become pure clear energy. They are rotated outwards and draw my extended arms further out behind me, and up. Just a brief moment. A moment of clear energy. Fresh. Both warm and cool. Full and empty.

Now, as my movement comes to a close, I am standing with my hands out in front of me, fingers gesturing upwards. I smile. My heart feels light and joyful.

Opening my eyes, I see the oak tree on the horizon, with its many arms lifted, fine fingers of branches emerging out of the dense heart of ivy and reaching directly upwards. I feel my own joy and lightness is witnessed through the gesture of the tree, reflecting my own gesture back to me.

> *Dancing tree. I know my connection to this tree, and bow in greeting. We are the same. I smile again as I recognise this. I feel she could be smiling back at me, and laughing.*
>
> (Excerpt from my Authentic Movement journal)

As Merlin Sheldrake writes, "[L]ook at the network, and it starts to look back at you." (2020: 240)

Here I am called to look again at the myth of *Inanna, Sumerian Queen of Heaven and Earth* (Wolkstein & Kramer 1983), a story which has inspired and guided me for many decades (Hartley 2001). Inanna travels to the Underworld to meet her dark sister Ereshkigal. She listens to 'the Great Below', to the Earth body and all it holds, and is impelled to journey there to pay witness to her sister's suffering. In the act of listening, journeying to meet Ereshkigal and witnessing her pain, Inanna brings consciousness to her sister's suffering. Now, in another turn of the spiral of this myth's development, I imagine Ereshkigal as an expression of Earth consciousness, suffering in darkness for so long but now awakening as Inanna, as we, begin to listen and to see with empathy and compassion. Inanna bears witness to the birth pains of awakening consciousness, as a reciprocal relationship of deep listening between human and Earth is re-awakened. Ereshkigal, as the once-silent voice of Earth body, cries out and we must hear.

Dancing with Earth Consciousness

> *My body moving is how Earth dances – I am an expression of Earth's creative energy.*
>
> (Excerpt from my Authentic Movement journal)

I often have the feeling that some mysterious presence – Spirit, the soul of Gaia perhaps – is expressing *through me* in my Authentic Movement practice. Waiting for me to simply turn up and open my awareness to what may want to arise and express, it moves through me, shaping my body into gestures, patterns, mudras, stillness and sometimes sound. Energy playing with me, through me. My bodily form responding. There may be no sense of content that my mind can grasp – no story or image to anchor the experience within my personal history, or even within a collective and cultural store of myths and memories. My body, formed from the elements of Earth, becomes a vessel for the expression of Spirit in such moments. Insight and meaning might arise, but they might not. I am asked to simply be present, an open vessel for the movement of Spirit through me, and into the world. Such moments are profound gifts. They carry healing energy, integrating me once again into the fabric of life so that my small concerns and worries, the pain in my body and the hurt in my heart, can all be safely held, and even laid to rest for a while, within a mystery much larger than they are.

> *I am following flowing pathways of energy, enjoying the movement. The feeling of being 'an expression of Gaia' arises. It invites a feeling of beauty to flow through me – from my feet to my fingers. I am filled with Gaia's beauty.*
>
> (Excerpt from my Authentic Movement journal)

When I experience my body as a vessel in this way, I feel in direct relationship with this presence that expands my awareness beyond the familiar boundaries of my individual self, my physical body, my personal history and my ordinary human limitations. I move closer to a feeling of at-oneness with both Earth and Spirit, knowing them to be married in the knotty sinews and fluid meanderings of my body. *Conscious body* is born in the meeting with *conscious Earth*.

> *Lying on my belly, head lifted and hands tucked under my throat and upper chest, folded in. Tail lifts, back arches softly, forelegs on the floor ground me. My pelvic floor opens. I am vessel. I feel the possibility of Earth energy and Sky energy moving through me, meeting within me. There is something unknown, mysterious here. I wait. Simply present, listening.*
>
> "Lie on your belly on the Earth", Earth tells me.
>
> (Excerpt from my Authentic Movement journal)

The experience that Nature is not only a recipient of our attention, our attentive listening and appreciative gaze, but is also listening to and watching us, is woven into the worldview of indigenous peoples. David Abram writes:

> *Such deference in the face of natural elements – the clear sense that the animate terrain is not just speaking to us but also listening to us – bears out Merleau-Ponty's thesis of perceptual reciprocity; to listen to*

> *the forest is also, primordially, to feel oneself listened to by the forest, just as to gaze at the surrounding forest is to feel oneself exposed and visible, to feel oneself watched by the forest.* (Abram 1997, 2017: 153)

In coming to the experience of body as vessel, the feeling of body as offering naturally arises. The conscious body, connected with the *web of life*, with Earth and Spirit, becomes an offering. Embodied presence becomes an act of service to Gaia.

From Tribe to Individual to Interbeing

> *Vitally, the human race is dying. It is like a great uprooted tree, with its roots in the air. We must plant ourselves again in the universe."*
> — *D.H. Lawrence*

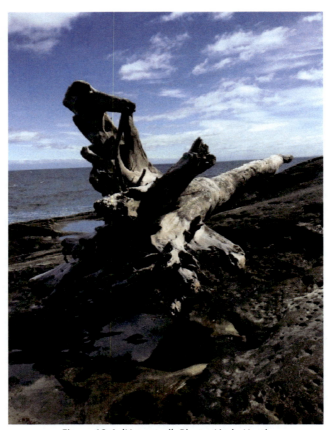

Figure 12.4: 'Uprooted'. Photo: Linda Hartley

Today in many indigenous cultures the sense of collective identity is still strong. Some traditional Asian cultures, perhaps rooted in religions such as Buddhism, also tend towards a stronger sense of collective identity and responsibility than modern westernised cultures with a strong drive towards individualism. They give the wellbeing of the whole, which includes the natural world that they inhabit, precedence over the individual's wishes and needs. These peoples understand that the individual cannot survive and flourish outside of a healthy community and environment, so care of the greater whole is of paramount importance. Interbeing has always been a foundation of human society, but we have lost touch with this during our quest of the individual. A sense of separation, isolation and weakened psychic foundations can be the result.

Having trodden the path of individuation and developed what must have been an essential step in our evolution in times past, we have undoubtedly reached a turning point. We cannot go further on the path of separation without wreaking irreparable damage – upon ourselves, individually and collectively, and upon our environment. We are seeing the signs of this everywhere in the world. The turn of the spiral of the evolution of consciousness requires that we re-embrace the sense of Interbeing, but now with the gift of consciousness that the age of individuation has enabled. To me this is an extraordinarily exciting step, one which brings gratitude for the privilege of being alive at this time and able to participate in such a transition.

Our sense of personal boundary or interface develops within the culture in which we grow up, is informed by it, and will determine how we contribute to that culture as we grow into adults. As explored earlier, the permeability or rigidity of cellular membranes influences and reflects the quality of psychological boundaries that maintain the integrity of self. This also has bearing upon our quality and depth of openness to the invisible realms of Spirit, the Sacred within and around us. In cultures where a shared collective identity is strong, the embrace of Interbeing, a receptivity to connection with others, might lead to an enhanced openness to connection with Other. More fluid, transparent, permeable or expanded personal boundaries reveal pathways to the experience of Spirit.

From my embodied explorations of embryonic life, and witnessing others on this journey, I learn that in the womb we are close to Spirit: our membranous boundaries and the umbilical cord which grows from them are sensitive and permeable to the mother-universe which holds us. A primarily positive experience in the womb allows these membranes to remain open in a healthy and responsive way – places of connection, communication and transformation, as well as protection. This supports the capacity to feel connected to the *web of life* whilst also feeling safe and held.

As we move through the spiral of life and arrive fully grown as adults, the quality of our boundaries once again becomes important if we choose, or are impelled, to turn towards spiritual unfolding. As explored earlier, during the journey through childhood the invisible realms retreat into the background for most, as the physical and psychological challenges of growing are mastered. Then come the eruptions of adolescence where aspects of the Dynamic Ground are felt to surge up again. In early adulthood the new challenges of finding our place in the world, developing a career, raising a family, discovering our unique contribution to society might demand all our resources. At some point on the spiral of growth, and often (though not always) after these earlier challenges have been met well enough, attention might turn towards developing the spiritual life.

For the person born into an indigenous society where self is identified in relation to the collective, spiritual life might have been central throughout their growing up. For those of us who have grown up in more individualistic cultures, with a sense of self defined by our own personal boundaries and achievements rather than those of our family, tribe and land, opening again to Spirit and the *web of life*, which we had some knowing of in the womb, might be fraught with new challenges. We need each other in this quest – a teacher, a sangha, an embodied sense of our Interbeing, our deep-rooted connection and interdependence with other beings, human and more-than-human. Deepening our relationship with Earth, opening our sensitivity to her presence, needs and gifts, becomes our support in this work. Opening to a *sense* of belonging to the collective of beings, and to all of life, offers a path towards *experiencing* at-oneness with the Sacred.

Reginald Ray writes:

> *When we begin to inhabit the body as our primary way of sensing, feeling, and knowing the world, when our thought operates as no more than a handmaiden of that somatic way of being, then we find that we as human beings are in a state of intimate relationship and connection with all that is.* (Ray 2014: 24)

In recognising our intimate interconnectedness, we also become more sensitively attuned to the health and sickness of our environment, of Earth and Nature. We might feel that the problems that afflict our world are reflected in our own health issues, both personal and collective. Many parallels can be drawn between the global epidemics of cancer, stress and immunological disorders, heart disease, viral contagion, digestive disorders, and so on. If we look closely into the symptoms of our own ill-health we can find reflections of the state of our planet's health too.

After one particular movement session this prayer came spontaneously to me:

> *Dear Mother Earth*
>
> *Where you are wounded, my own body resonates with your pain. May the loving care, attention and healing I give to my body also help to heal your body, precious Earth body.*
>
> *And where we humans have hurt and decimated you, and you in your wisdom and intelligence have revived, healed and become abundant again, may we humbly learn from you how to heal ourselves.*

Climate Change as Symptom

> *Climate change is the simple consequence of forgetting the holiness of this mysterium in which we're bodily immersed.* (Abram 2020)

> *The reanimation of our world is crucial to ecological healing. If we live in the perception that the world is dead, we will inevitably kill what is alive.* (Eisenstein 2018: 266)

As Abram and Eisenstein so eloquently argue, climate change is a symptom and a factor but not the cause of degradation of life on Earth (2018: 80-82). All systems of Gaia are ailing because of human activity, weakening the life of Earth, slowly killing it. Human activity has been damaging the natural ecosystems of Earth for centuries, but this has accelerated since the industrial revolution and ramped up to dangerous levels in the 20th and 21st centuries.

We need to heal all aspects of living Gaia, restore natural ecosystems so that once again they can sustain the rich diversity of planetary life. Restoring a sustainable climate is part of this; so is ceasing our invasive intrusions into the wilds, where we upset natural ecosystems, endanger plant, animal and human lives, and bring new diseases from wild animals into our midst. And in parallel with this is the need to restore natural health within the human population, to minimise the need for expensive and sometimes risky or toxic medical procedures by attending to the restoration of wellness. I am not denying the amazing gifts of modern medicine and surgery, but before a situation becomes critical or an emergency, often we can first seek health through living in greater harmony with the natural world, moderating our desires and our activity, turning to natural and preventative medicine when we can, and living closer to the rhythms and the needs of our own nature. Stress compromises the health of our nervous, immune and endocrine systems, as well as putting pressure on our heart, breathing, digestion and indeed all physical and psychological functions. It is the same with Earth – when we keep adding stresses to the delicate balance of ecosystems, somewhere that balance will begin to fail and ecological sickness and collapse will result.

We know that human activity has damaged the ozone layer, the protective mantle that shields Earth from too much harmful radiation. In the same way we individuals have a protective energetic membrane that surrounds us[3]. I imagine it as a reflection of the amniotic sac which contained us *in utero*, a non-material imprint of the layer of protection we first created for ourselves in the womb. When we are not in good health, psychologically as well as physically, this membrane can be felt to be weak or damaged, perhaps too permeable, just as the ozone layer has become damaged as the health of planet Earth has deteriorated. We are a microcosm of the greater body that is Gaia.

Climate change is a symptom of the wider disruption of natural ecosystems, just as severe covid is a symptom of the disruption of natural balance within the human body; this virus has been found to have a talent for seeking out our vulnerabilities and weaknesses and inflaming them into more extreme illness. Both our human and planetary health are crying out for us to attend to deeper causes, to listen to what is out of balance, in excess, contaminated, stripped of genuine nourishment and loving care. We are now at the turning point where we can, indeed must, choose to change this.

Despite the all-too-often destructive power humans have been able to exert over Nature, Mary-Jayne Rust reminds us that:

> [C]limate change and the ecological crisis are like an act of Nature rising up, showing humans who is in charge, offering our dominant culture an opportunity for a collective rite of passage. Facing our own extinction could be seen as the Mother of all Rites of Passage for Western civilisation. (Rust 2020: 27)

Any efforts we make towards healing and transforming our own elements – the water, air, earth, fire and space within us – are part of the healing of Gaia, as we are not separate. As we take steps to create greater balance and wellness within, we are adding a drop in the ocean of healing that Gaia needs. Every drop is important, every drop counts. Our own healing affects the whole, is part of the whole. At those times when all we are able to attend to is our personal wellbeing and health, we can dedicate this to collective and planetary healing.

> [W]e enrich and deepen our experience of self through our capacity to identify with others – other humans as well as other species. Through this we can feel compassion and empathy for the other and a sense of ecological identity (Naess, 1988) …
>
> The ecological self is inextricably linked with, and embedded in, the rest of nature. (Rust 2020: 67)

Love, reverence, respect, care for sacred Earth is required of us to heal the problems we face. Going beyond what we know, despairing, giving up, then giving over to, we come to an empty place where new solutions can emerge that are based on love, not scientific engineering and more 'progress' – which often create as many problems as they solve – or attempts to suppress the problem as humans have been doing for so long.

In this great work of our time we need to hold all injustices as part of one whole – ecological and environmental, social, racial, sexual, political and economic. This complex tapestry that is life on Earth is calling out to be re-woven into something of beauty, vitality and sustainability once again. The somatic practice of embodied awareness has gifts to offer in this work.

13: Collective Body

In earlier chapters we explored the development of the individual human being – as implanting embryo, infant and child – and the inherent need and orientation to seek personal connection and relationship that is fundamental to being human. Connection with others is essential for healthy development and ongoing wellbeing, both physical and psychological.

And we have looked into the connectivity within the individual body, and of the individual in relation to the Earth body and the whole of Nature.

In a turn of the spiral, we may also come into deepened *conscious* relationship with our community of fellow humans and with the Sacred, as our awareness expands to embrace more of who we are, of our potential and of the world we inhabit. Describing the practice of Tibetan Buddhist Yoga, Reginald Ray writes of the three *yanas*, or 'vehicles', stages of spiritual development:

> *Hinayana primarily addresses our own physical body, what we may term the "personal body"; Mahayana speaks of the larger, interpersonal dimension of our somatic being, which we may designate the "interpersonal body"; and Vajrayana speaks about our body in its largest, most universal dimensions, which we may call the "cosmic body".* (Ray 2014: 255)
>
> *The cosmic body is the primordial "body" of the earth, of the natural world and its nonhuman creatures, of which we are ... embodiments and expressions.* (Ray 2014: 130)

The Discipline of Authentic Movement offers a space to explore conscious embodied connection, with self, with one other, with a group of others, with the wider environment we dwell within, and with the numinous, in ever-increasing circles of inclusivity. Janet Adler has given the name the Collective Body (2002) to experiences of and within these expanding and deepening circles of connectivity. Earlier in the evolution of the Discipline she developed forms such as the Long Circle to support the exploration of embodied participation in the collective. She writes:

> *The longing to be seen by another and to see another open toward a longing to participate within a whole, to discover one's relationship to many without losing an authentic or truthful awareness of oneself, without betraying oneself…*
>
> *… Readiness for a larger group reflects a growing awareness of a desire to belong. Exploration of such a longing opens individuals toward questions of the relationship between the self and the collective. The embodiment of collective consciousness can only become manifest because of the embodiment of personal consciousness.* (Adler 2002: 108-9)

Here Adler speaks of the need to be grounded in the 'personal body', to have done enough work within our somatic and psychological being so that our inner witness is clear and strong enough to stay present within a collective of individuals each exploring their place within the whole. Although we all live within a collective or 'interpersonal body', as Ray names it, we do this in a largely unconscious way for much of the time. With training and practice though, we can develop the capacity for conscious embodiment of the collective. In Discipline of Authentic Movement circles we track the expressions of each individual, and also open awareness to the unfolding of relationship and connection between them and with the space they inhabit. As movers and witnesses open in these ways, and come together after a movement circle to share experiences, consciousness of the movement of the collective body grows. The circle becomes a sacred space where intimacy and connection – the individual within the collective – can be nurtured.

Adler goes on to say:

> *If we abandon such essential ground by sacrificing or manipulating the personal voice in order to feel as though we belong, we do not truly belong, we are not truly whole. And if we ignore the opportunity for consciously embodied membership we heighten our sense of alienation, isolation, and despair, all of which insidiously and profoundly disable us as individuals.* (Adler 2002: 108-9)

It is important to stress that we do not move away from – above or beyond – the personal as we begin to encounter experiences of collective embodiment or the mystical dimensions of practice. The personal – our histories, memories, psychological conditioning and embodied patterning – is the way into exploration of other realms. Sometimes felt as a portal into the Sacred, the personal dimension of practice is eventually realised as not separate from, but integrally woven within the Sacred. The personal and transpersonal meet and support each other when both are given space and attention, when both are invited to unfold into conscious awareness.

Janet's research led her to continue to develop the work within the collective, as subtler levels of experience began to emerge more frequently amidst circles of movers and witnesses. As the energetic, subtle, sacred, or mystical began to reveal itself more fully, new forms that could invite and support these unfoldings became apparent. The Ritual Practice is one such form: we begin with the 'declaring circle', where the participants stand in a circle around the edge of the empty space, witnessing the empty space and taking a moment to connect to their readiness to move or be a witness. Each in turn declares their intention and makes eye contact with each other person. Once all have declared and committed to being either a mover or a witness for this period of practice, witnesses sit, the bell sounds, and movers enter the space to begin the 'moving and witnessing circle'. At the end of an agreed period of time, and after a short transition, the 'speaking and listening circle' begins, where each mover in turn speaks in as much depth and detail as they are able of a specific moment of their movement; each other participant can respond as a moving witness, external speaking witness, listening or integral witness, offering something of their own experience of the named moment. In this way a fuller and deeper sense of the moment is created, as each person affirms their participation in the collective-becoming-conscious.

In my experience, this practice integrates the three 'yanas' that Ray describes: it supports the intimacy of dyadic work between one mover and one witness, where exploration of personal material is given as much space as is needed, and brings this into the collective; each mover and each witness comes into deepening connection with each other mover and witness, and so a collective of conscious individuals can develop. The experience of each individual is significant, is honoured, explored, shared, witnessed by each other individual in the circle. This makes the Discipline quite unique. As subtler experiences of Spirit arise and are shared in these ways, spiritual practice becomes a truly conscious collective phenomenon.

Discussing ritual in *The Wild Edge of Sorrow*, Francis Weller writes:

> *Simply said, ritual is any gesture done with emotion and intention by an individual or a group that attempts to connect the individual or the community with transpersonal energies for the purposes of healing and transformation. Ritual is the pitch through which the personal and collective voices of our longing and creativity are extended to the unseen dimensions of life, beyond our conscious minds and into the realms of nature and spirit.* (Weller 2015: 76)

As the "voices of our longing and creativity are extended to the unseen dimensions of life", we begin to feel our participation extend beyond the collective or 'interpersonal body' to what Ray names the 'cosmic body'. Direct knowing of our interweaving within the *web of life* arises in spontaneous moments: we might feel our connection with Earth and Nature, our ancestors, animal spirits, pure energy, or the vast spaciousness of the Universe; we might be moved by moments of profound joy or love or gratitude, or indeed awe and fear; and we share such experiences within a collective that is becoming conscious. Becoming at-one with all we are capable of being conscious of in that moment, what Janet calls *unitive consciousness* arises – not separate, not alone, not merged, but deeply embedded within the whole as consciousness, as Spirit embodied.

Communication and Connection

Communication and connection between participants of the collective body occur in increasingly subtle ways: from the sensory and verbal, which are tangible expressions and more readily understood through our knowing about anatomy, physiology and reflective thought processes, the mysteries of non-verbal, non-sensory connectivity begin to arise. Often there is a sense of dwelling within a shared field of energy and an intelligence that moves through one person, then another, or several at one time. The very space comes alive and takes on qualities of its own, as might specific locations in the studio. Without conscious awareness that is mediated through the familiar sensory or cognitive channels, and with eyes closed, the movers nevertheless seem to 'know' where the other is and what they are doing. I am reminded of the mycorrhizal networks connecting trees, allowing them to communicate with each other, invisible beneath the ground. Magic happens.

Synchronicities occur, timing is important. There might be moments of mirroring a shared gesture, of arriving in the exact place in space another mover previously occupied and repeating the exact same gesture; or energy might move powerfully through one mover while others seem to 'hold' or 'anchor' the mover through their still presence, before the energy moves on and through another mover. Here are a few small moments amongst many small moments which, together, weave an experience of subtle connectivity:

> *Two movers stand with eyes closed, facing each other across the empty space. They gesture simultaneously with their hands, held out to their sides and a little in front, palms facing upwards. One brings thumbs and middle fingers to touch; the other holds her palms open. A silent conversation begins.*
>
> *Later, simultaneously they come down to lie on the floor, on their backs. One rests the fingertips of her left hand lightly on the left side of her upper chest. The other reaches her left hand over to rest her open palm on her right upper chest. Her right hand then moves down to rest on her solar plexus.*

* * * * *

> *Another day – both movers come to lie on their backs at the same moment, both with arms spread wide. One has both feet on the floor, knees up; the other rests one foot on the floor and extends the other leg. At precisely the same moment both lift their left hand slightly off the floor and pause. Then one continues her journey upwards with the hand; the other lets her hand rest back on the floor.*

* * * * *

> *Two movers lie on their backs. One extends her left hand far out along the floor, palm facing upwards; I recognise a gesture of receptivity, of inviting contact. The other mover extends her leg up into the air until her foot is directly above the open palm. I anticipate connection. After some time they finally meet, and following some initial exploration the hand is finally holding the foot, full and warm contact.*

* * * * *

> *A mover is birthing something powerful, creaturely, more-than-human – energy deep in the belly, rising up deep into the throat. She labours. Another mover stands in complete stillness. Her left forearm is held out and parallel to the floor, fingers curled around into a loose fist. The forearm takes on deepened presence and becomes an anchor, anchored in this specific place in space. The space between the two movers becomes alive, a web of energy connecting them.*

Shortly after witnessing and writing about this last moment, I came across Robin Wall Kimmerer's description of *Braiding Sweetgrass* where she tells how:

> [T]he sweetest way is to have someone else hold the end so that you pull gently against each other, all the while leaning in ... one holding steady while the other shifts the slim bundles over one another, each in its turn. Linked by sweetgrass, there is reciprocity between you, linked by sweetgrass, the holder as vital as the braider.
> (Kimmerer 2013: ix)

I felt I had witnessed a similar sacred ritual, expressed through the medium of conscious bodies moving in the studio space – an ancient rite performed by women coming into sacred relationship with each other and with the natural world. As I reflect on this process, I begin to see many other examples of such sacred bonds between people, where one holds still and anchors another's movement of profound transition or deep journeying. A midwife holding steady as the mother labours to give birth; the priest or priestess standing firmly in sacred time and space as the couple cross the threshold into a new life together; or the spiritual midwife who keeps vigil at the end of a life, as the dying person crosses the final threshold. Sacred passage calls for this service of the one who holds steady, who anchors, witnesses and mediates the moment.

The question of how we sense the movement of energy in our own body, and in the space between and around movers, is one that fascinates me. Through which channels of perception do we sense energy and connection when eyes are closed and there is no audible sound or physical contact? When ways of knowing do not appear to be mediated through the physical pathways of nerves and sensory organs, how do we know what is happening across the space and beyond? Through skin, cellular awareness, subtle energetic sense organs and pathways that are not to be found in western anatomy books? In this practice we are learning to discern between intuitive knowing that relies upon all of our senses and more, and projection which arises through the filter of our personal history, our conditioning and prejudices. It is in the speaking and listening circle, after moving and witnessing, that the difference can be clarified and clear intuitive knowing brought into consciousness. This is the collective body becoming conscious.

Within the individual body it might be that a fullness is sensed in some particular location, or we notice a movement has already begun and attention goes there; as described in an earlier chapter, attention increases the presence and flow of energy, and this initiates movement if we allow it. The potential for moving with the flows of energy through and around us is always present, but for most of the time we do not perceive these potentials for movement. When we are open to, and allow them, we can feel that a presence, an intelligence greater than our 'small self' is guiding us: "I am moved", as Mary Starks Whitehouse discovered (1963: 53)

Within the collective body it might be that we can sense, by some as yet uncharted function, the fullness of energy in a particular part of the space – in a mover or in the space between movers. Or the energetic ripples coming from another's movement might reach us across the space. Opening awareness and giving attention to such phenomena would surely support those movements across and through the space to unfold, even when a mover remains still and present, a silent anchor and energetic witness of the collective body. At the growing edge of collective consciousness, where consciousness of the collective body is expanding, movers and witnesses may feel that they are participating in what is unfolding in subtle ways, even though they are not directly engaged with the movement that is stirring the energetic space.

The practice named by Janet as Ceremony, as well as the Ritual Practice, supports such explorations of energy and consciousness moving within the collective. Subtle expressions of intuitive knowing can be cultivated through these practices (Adler, Morrissey and Sager 2022).

In the following example I take the liberty of adding my own perspective as witness of both the group's movement and also their sharing at the start of the retreat (with their permission). We meet after nearly sixteen months of enduring the anxieties, fears, frustrations and collective trauma of the pandemic; participants bring much stress, emotion and exhaustion with them into the space, some of it from their personal lives, some of it from the wider field. At one point I witness a moment when the individual journeys seem to settle into a collective stillness; later they will acknowledge their shared experience of connection in this moment:

> *Towards the end of the moving time one mover sits and opens her throat, head tilts back slightly, mouth opens a little, slowly drinking in air. There is a deep silence in the room. Each mover has arrived, on the floor. Each has landed, their body surrendered to gravity, lying in various positions that suggest letting go or falling or simply being stopped.*
>
> *I feel I am witnessing a battlefield, after the battle is over, survivors and the wounded recognising, awakening to their situation, quietly attending to wounds. My story. But I hear in the speaking circle how much they each carry, and I witness how much the collective trauma that is in the wider field has impinged upon their personal embodiment. Here they can give expression to this and allow the knots to begin to unravel.*
>
> *I pray that each may find healing here, and as the retreat unfolds, I see from open smiling faces and expanded gestures that they do. Pain is transformed as it is felt, embodied in movement and witnessed within the collective of movers and witnesses.*

Embryonic Roots of Embodied Relational Spiritual Practice

In an earlier chapter I made the bold statement that all we will grow into and experience in life, including the foundations of our own style of relational patterning, is already present during gestation in the womb, embodied in gesture and form as the embryo develops. Now I do not know this as a scientifically proven fact, though we do know that our DNA contains all our potential from the very moment of conception; which traits will actually come into expression depends to some extent on environmental conditions, the 'invitations' that come to us as we meet the world and grow.

However, my study of embryology through reading about the process and contemplating images, as well as my own experiences of embodying the gestures of the embryo and witnessing the experiences of many students and clients over the years, has supported an intuitive 'knowing' that the roots of all we will become are present from our embryonic days, just waiting for the right conditions in order to become fully embodied and expressed.

I would like to suggest that the experience of the collective body has also been known to us (though not quite in the conscious way I have been discussing above) from our early time in the womb, held, contained and witnessed by our mother-womb-world. Mother's body is the embryo and foetus's world, the ground which mediates all of the elements of the material world and the beings and events it contains. Through the experience of being held closely within the womb space, the embryo begins to know connection to all that exists in the world. Through mother's body, her emotions, thoughts and energy, the vibrations of the world she inhabits reach the tiny being growing inside her.

As we have explored, the pre-embryo begins to secure his place in the womb-world by creating a two-layered protective and nurturing membrane around himself, formed out of his own cellular self. This membrane intimately connects with a third layer that is part of the lining of the mother's womb. Here, direct experience of connection is known, one being meeting the boundaries of another. This is our first direct knowing of another's physical presence, occurring as implantation takes place and evolving as the placenta is formed. Within this meeting of embryonic and maternal membranes I suggest that an embryonic experience of self-coming-into-relationship-with-other occurs. Perhaps the seed of the inner witness – the capacity to witness one's own experience – and of the outer witness – the capacity to witness another clearly –- is planted at this earliest stage of a new life.

One flowering of this seed might occur as the conscious awareness of a circle of witnesses in Authentic Movement practice touches the conscious awareness of the movers, reflecting the meeting of embryonic membranes with maternal membranes as the womb's three-layered container is formed. In this meeting of the inner witness of each mover with the attentive presence of each outer witness, the potential to 'know' expands to include so much more than the immediate experience of each individual. The meeting place acts as a conduit, a portal for other realms of experience to become known, beyond all that is immediately visible.

Global Expressions of Embodied Relational Spiritual Practice

There are many other group practices that might help cultivate a sense of collective presence and awareness. Meditation for example, which offers the space for practitioners to self-reflect and contemplate deeply, when practised by a group repeatedly over time can engender deep feelings of connection and belonging. Meditators come to know themselves as a *sangha*, a community of practitioners who share beliefs, aspirations and a deep and subtle sense of connectedness, of *Interbeing* with each other and all of life. A spiritual or religious community of any persuasion can hold this potential for deep belonging, which goes beyond the obvious social ties that support members in tangible ways. A shared practice where each participant is encountering their inner self with compassion and authentic feeling can offer experiences of deep belonging and support collective consciousness to emerge. My own experience of being embedded in a community practising the ancient art of T'ai Chi Ch'uan gave me a first taste of this through embodied practice. Through meditation, Authentic Movement, dance, community singing and other shared practices I have also come to experience a deepened sense of connection.

During the period of extended pandemic lockdowns, I took up some of the opportunities to join with online groups practising meditation, and within the field of *subtle* or *sacred activism*. There are many such groups all around the globe, which gives me some hope during those days when the news seems filled with only darkness and despair. One such practice, the *GaiaTree Circle* offered by David Nicol and Kate Naga as an online practice space, supports a global community to develop[1]. The guided meditations explicitly invite participants to bring awareness together to create a shared energetic field, which is focused towards personal, collective and planetary healing. Meeting a group of people online, often thousands of miles apart, can potentially feel like a not-fully-embodied experience, but they have developed a sensing practice that brings each participant's immediate sensory and energetic experience into relationship with others. Such practices can guide us towards the experience of a conscious collective body where we might find connection, strength and healing – for ourselves, each other, Earth and Nature. Nicol writes of his work:

> *This traditional view [of mystical practice] is giving way in our times to a rising spiritual sensibility that seeks to connect all the parts and dimensions of life with each other. Where the focus is on developing new and deeper capacities of relational intelligence that allow us to heal the wounds that have separated us from each other and the wider community of life.*
>
> *With this emerging sensibility, the goal of our spiritual activities is changing. Instead of understanding our spiritual work primarily as an inner, private, individual journey toward Source-realization or unity consciousness, the focus is shifting to the development of relational fields with emergent creative capacities and healing powers that serve not only personal but also cultural and collective transformation. The spiritual goal of this emerging era could be conceived as a more embodied, pragmatic, and distributed realization of unity consciousness, manifesting throughout our personal, social, economic, and political lives. The inner and outer realms are coming closer together, as are the personal and the collective.* (Nicol 2020: online)

Some other expressions of this movement include the Global Joy Summit, evolving from the teachings of His Holiness the Dalai Lama and Reverend Desmond Tutu[2], and the Collective Trauma Healing work of Thomas Hubl[3]. For many decades Thich Nhat Hanh has been a guiding light in the practice of developing *Interbeing* within communities, Earth and Nature through meditation, engaged Buddhism and the nurturing of sangha[4].

I am sure there was a time when this intuitive way of knowing was more readily available to more people. In a long-distant past there must have been an increased collective capacity for sensitivity to the subtle realms; the knowing and knowledge, insight and wisdom, accessed by spiritual practitioners, shamans, yogis and the innovators of traditional healing systems such as Traditional Chinese Medicine and Ayurveda suggests this. As receptivity to such practices grows today, may we hope that a time is coming when such awareness and sensitivity is again becoming more accessible to more people. The need and the longing to experience love, respect and care for the collective body of humanity, Earth and Nature is deep and pressing.

Part 5

Endings and Beginnings

14: Transparency and the Aging Body

During a lifetime there will inevitably be times when we feel more connected and less connected to Spirit. Sometimes it may feel so distant, so inaccessible that we fear we have lost connection altogether. From the development of the embryo, foetus and child when Spirit is becoming securely embodied, and on through a whole life cycle we spiral around the core tasks of being true to self, respectful of the needs of others, and humble in the presence of the Sacred. The spiral path takes us, many times, cycling around the tasks of integration within our personality and relationships in the world, and impels us to travel both inwards and out beyond our known and limited sense of self. Sometimes we are deeply challenged when Spirit is wounded, tired or completely hidden from view. The journey in and down on the path of descent and *endarkenment*, as well as up and beyond on the path of ascent and *enlightenment* are both called for on the path of awakening consciousness.

When we feel the blessing of being fully embodied, mind present within the body, no separation, no observing self, then we may arrive into feelings of deep peace. Joy, love, awe, gratitude for life and the blessings of Nature might arise, or a gentle bliss that permeates all levels of being – body, sensations, feelings; mind, soul, cells – all are washed through with these feelings. They will not last forever, cannot be held onto, but are moments that show us the way towards greater peace and harmony with all of life, within us and in the world around us.

Embodied awareness practices such as somatic movement and Authentic Movement offer ways to explore and taste the pleasures and joys of living in a sensing, feeling body. The joys often come through experiences of suffering and pain, through travelling into the dark recesses of our unconscious life to uncover buried emotions, memories, lost parts of ourselves, as well as hidden treasures. Movement can encourage the flow of energy in the body, which evokes pleasurable sensations; it can trigger endorphins that engender feelings of happiness and bliss in the body[1]. And there is more – a consciously embodied sense of self can be awakened, bringing feelings such as clarity, confidence, groundedness, connection, presence; the soul is touched, opening us to the treasures hidden within the heart of our being; and Spirit may be experienced directly, awakening, expanding and transforming consciousness towards wholeness and connection with the Universal.

Movement and dance have been integral to the cultural and spiritual life of people since ancient times: the yogi and yogini find deep inner peace and balance through the practice of yoga; the whirling Dervish surrenders to ecstasy as she spins into the still point at the centre; shamans and indigenous communities worldwide communicate with spirits and ancestors through ritual dance; the master of T'ai Chi Ch'uan finds the delicate balance of stillness within movement and movement within stillness; a classical Indian dancer embodies the stories of the gods and goddesses through exquisitely tuned gestures; and in more recent times, the youth of all cultures find joy in the dances of their generation, be it jive, salsa, the Charleston, tango, hip hop, and so many more. Each community, each era finds its own expression of raw energy through dance and movement, secular or sacred, where emotions can be expressed, the joy of moving experienced, and sometimes Spirit touched.

Of course, it has not always been like this. Western and some eastern cultures have gone through centuries of suppression, denial and denigration of the body; spiritual and religious beliefs have judged physical expression and dance in particular to be sinful, and there are still cultures today where such beliefs are held, especially in relation to women's bodies. But alongside this there have always been rebellious or 'subversive' elements of culture where the joy of movement and the pleasures of embodied life have held sway. The power of such natural expressions cannot be suppressed forever.

Spirit Grows Younger as Body Ages

It was some years ago that I remember sharing with a group of colleagues, during one of those rich and rambling conversations, that I felt my Spirit growing younger as I aged. At the time I was not yet truly in my elder years but I could feel them nudging closer. One woman told me that according to Native American traditions this is how it should rightly be – Spirit grows younger as Body ages. I think again of the experience of transparency that consciously embodied movement practice can cultivate. In those moments when the 'density of personal history' – embedded in our cells and tissues as memories, emotions, resistance, psychological and physical patterns – clears enough to allow the light within us to shine through, the invisible becomes visible, no longer obscured. Many years of embodied awareness practice might support this transformation from density to transparency. It might arrive in moments of grace, or be a gradual and constant path of evolution towards something stable and enduring.

When I was younger, I imagined the potential of elderhood to be an arrival in a place of greater wisdom and contentment! Now I see this was perhaps a little naïve. Certainly, we hope to become wiser as we age. And there can be the contentment of knowing and appreciating what has been experienced and achieved, knowing that it is not necessary to keep on striving and achieving in many areas of life and work. This can be a relief and a source of joy and contentment if we can accept the arrival. For some, contentment might come with the delights of grandparenting, the simple pleasures of tending a garden, the satisfaction of having completed some work, big or small, that has contributed in some way to others, to community, to the Earth or whatever we hold most dear. Spirit can feel lighter as we let go of old burdens and responsibilities we no longer need to carry, and some elders may embody a quality of translucence with this lightening of the load. But aging is also, for most, a time of increasing physical weakness, illness, maybe disability, pain and discomfort. There are new journeys to be made in order to truly arrive into the wisdom, contentment and maybe even joy of elderhood, and not all of us will complete this journey. Acceptance and surrender will be called for. The capacity to hold both the Light and the Dark simultaneously – not oscillating between them as perhaps we have been doing all our lives, but embracing both at once – is one of the challenges and potential gifts of our elder years.

The Buddha described the four existential sufferings of human life as 'birth, old age, sickness and death'. If we are fortunate enough not to die too young, and to have had opportunities to embody, learn and grow through some practice that cultivates presence, we may find we can arrive into older age with enough acceptance and grace to manage the pain and limitations it brings. The body becomes less resilient with age, less ready to recover from injury and illness; the dance between doing all we can to support our health and wellbeing, balanced with acceptance of what cannot be changed, becomes more intense, the edge between them sharper.

Combinations of genetic tendencies, psychological and social conditioning, environmental factors, illness and old injuries, opportunities, and all the uses and abuses we might put our bodies through during a long life inevitably affect how we age and how well our bodies recover from injury and illness. For many there comes a time when the aging of the body can feel at odds with the lightening of Spirit that is a potential gift of becoming older. When we are suffering the worst ravages that aging wreaks on the body we may feel completely cut off from Spirit. Janet Adler writes;

> *In the moment of suffering, the utter force of it fills the space so that awareness of anything other than the suffering is obliterated. Here we can know a separation from our source. It is in these moments, when we most need that very particular light of the numinous, that it may be inaccessible.* (Adler 2022: 319)

The practice of mindful attention, of being present in each moment, takes on a new imperative. When the body and the soul are in pain, or suffering in other ways, we will need to find ways to return to presence, being alert to the moments of potential beauty, joy and gratitude that might arise. A wise woman gave me the lovely phrase, 'little islands of pleasure and joy'. As my body ages and often gives me pain I need to attend to those tiny openings, potential portals into the wide embrace of Spirit that is actually always there, no matter what the body may be telling us – the cheerful yellow of the daffodils that opened today against a background of dark evergreens, spring's first warm breeze on my face, sunlight streaming through the rain on the windowpane, a baby's first smile. When I can no longer dance with joy or skip and run as I did when a child, I can still notice the small step I take with a certain amount of ease and grace, feeling a secure connection with Earth body once again. The sole of my foot touches the soul of the Earth, a momentary love affair. It will be hard to stay connected to these feelings when pain is insistent, but the little islands of pleasure and joy bring momentary relief and perhaps support the will to take the next small step.

Joyful Body, Painful Body

An infant and young child is potentially gifted with a magical existence in 'the garden of delight' (Washburn 2003:15) for the first two years or so of life. If the little one is fortunate to have a loving and caring enough environment to grow in, he can experience intense joy through the sensory and relational impressions that flood through him from his world. My nephew showed me a recent photo of his newborn son, just two months old, having a private smile to himself. In his eyes I saw the most stunning expression, which seemed to me to express sheer awe, love and delight – as if he was seeing something awesome, divine; joy and light were pouring from the little one's eyes. Of course, this is most likely my own projection, but we cannot but feel uplifted when we witness expressions of pure joy in a young being.

As we explored in earlier chapters, Spirit becomes embodied as the infant and young child learns to master his own body and interact with increasing degrees of agency within his environment. Joy might mark moments of personal achievement as each milestone of development is reached. We see the joy of movement in a child's play at its most intense as the capacity to become faster, stronger, more graceful, more vital grows. Children love to move, they need to move, they are learning through movement and they are expressing embodied Spirit with every gesture.

I know this was true for me. My happiest childhood memories are of running across green open fields, doing cartwheels on the beach, learning to skip, roller skate, jump the waves – and dance. The joy of movement has been the foundation of my life, though it was not until I was nineteen that I was bold enough to imagine I might be able to make some kind of career out of it! Parallel to this I had become interested in meditation but it took a long turn of the spiral before I was able to bring these two loves together, with my immersion in embodied awareness practices that enabled me to know again, now with more consciousness, the joyful body infused with Spirit.

I remember a specific moment, a few years ago:

> *I am sitting in my chair in the spacious studio where I had been leading Authentic Movement groups and other workshops for many years. A moment of transition between the moving and witnessing ritual, and the speaking and listening ritual. Participants of the retreat are moving about quietly, resting, making some notes or making tea. I look up through the skylight windows at the tall trees, swaying against a clear blue sky. Late spring, bright sunshine, gentle breeze, a perfect day. I am suddenly filled with utter joy and gratitude. Joy and gratitude for the light and bright space, not far from the sea, that has been home for my work for all these years; for the embrace of clear blue sky and ancient trees; for the beauty and uniqueness of each one of the wonderful people who have come to study and practice the Discipline of Authentic Movement with me, returning year after*

year to re-commit to this way of working; and joy and gratitude for all that is in my life at this moment and all that has led me here. I remember this as a perfect moment, a place to arrive, and even as I experienced it, I knew it could not be held onto.

Just a few months later everything changed, quite abruptly: my sister's cancer was diagnosed as terminal; events arose that meant I would not be able to continue working in this studio that had been my 'home' for many years; a beautiful retreat centre, close to beach, woods and marshes, that I had recently found was not going to be available anymore; and my mother's dementia took a swift decline as she felt unable to deal with my sister's prognosis. Many things began to unravel, the moment of joy was dissolving, and though I did not know it at the time I was facing another journey of descent. It was gradual, many steps down, much to be held and endured. My body carried the burden.

Just before the pandemic was confirmed I had already caught the coronavirus and processes of inflammation and pain in my body were escalated. This virus has a unique talent for searching out our individual weaknesses and vulnerabilities, so it can affect each of us differently. For me, enduring pain in joints and muscles has been the constant for more than three years; this is now recognised as one of the manifestations of 'long covid'. Naturally I have known physical injury and pain many times throughout my life as a mover and dancer, but in the past I have been able to manage it well enough through my movement practice, receiving bodywork, holistic therapies, sometimes rest or processing emotions that might lie beneath the physical symptoms. This was different. My body seemed to be aging more rapidly than I expected and the pain would not go away, the intensity of it moving from one place to another but a background pain always there.

Spirit calls differently when the body is in pain. Sometimes it calls us to become free of the physical body and truly dissolve into the Light. Like other longings we might have known, this comes from soul and needs to be heard. We can take the longing in a literal sense, wishing to be free of a body in pain once and for all. Or take it to mean something subtler – a call to search more deeply, follow the call of Spirit to find it once again in the dark and hidden places of the painful body. It is so often those times when we feel we are in the darkest places that we are in fact closest to Source, to the light of Spirit. When we can descend to the raw heart of our pain, the 'primary suffering' beneath the layers of 'secondary suffering' that we elaborate upon it, then an opening might appear. A tiny glimpse, a moment of spiritual comfort, or a full and direct connection again with Spirit, with our God, with an innate sense of wellness. It might come through inner voices or visions, the presence of ancestors, healers, deceased loved ones, inner guides or teachers. It might come through the sensation of a tender touch, a loving embrace, or a song.

I remember again the story of the woman walking along the beach and calling out to God – 'Why have you abandoned me at my time of greatest suffering?' And God speaks back to her – 'Do you not see one set of footsteps in the sand as you look back where you have travelled? This is where I carried you.' So we look deeper as we take another turn of the spiral, and if we are fortunate we can be surprised once again by the new life that waits to emerge. Like the spring bulbs pushing up faithfully each year out of the damp, dark soil.

Collectively we have seen an increase in both physical and mental health issues recently, not only directly related to covid-19 illness but as a result, I am sure, of the increased levels of stress and collective trauma that we have all had to endure. Here in the UK, we had the brutal fighting of the Brexit 'debate' that left our country on the verge of a collective nervous breakdown. Politics in the US was similarly tearing the fabric of society apart. And other countries had been facing the even more appalling horrors of war, persecution, climate disaster, acute poverty and famine. When the pandemic arrived out of this state of affairs, we were in a vulnerable place already; stress depletes the immune system so we were less able to resist the ravages of the virus. Then the daily diet of fear, restriction and isolation for many, and acute stress, loss and trauma for others, has undoubtedly led to further collective traumatisation and the undermining of our health. We should not be surprised that the collective body is suffering. Each person manifests this collective trauma in individual ways but we are all part of the whole, all connected in our sickness and health to one another.

When I can hold all of this within a wider embrace, I might ask – what is Spirit calling for, or calling forth? Deep and radical change is needed. Could all of this upheaval and trauma be the birth pangs of the new? Could it be the upsurging of forces from the Dynamic Ground, the Source of consciousness, demanding change, bringing change? As the individual body of each of us suffers, feels pain, breaks open, energy is surging into the collective and it might just bring the new life we are longing for and seeking. I see how the pain and illness of each individual body reflects some aspect of the collective body's pain, including that of the Earth body. As we work to heal our own broken bodies and minds, and to invite Spirit to shine through the cracks, we do this for the collective body too.

Healing and restoration, Clarissa Pinkola Estes tells us, are always possible. As long as we have the 'bone-seed', we have the 'key to life':

> *In myth and story, [bones] represent the indestructible soul-spirit. We know the soul-spirit can be injured, even maimed, but it is very nearly impossible to kill.*

> *You can dent the soul and bend it. You can hurt it and scar it, you can leave the marks of illness upon it, and the scorch marks of fear. But it does not die.* (1992: 35)

Indestructible Spirit lives through the cycles of life-death-rebirth and nothing is truly lost or wasted.

Coming Full Circle – Witnessing the Return to Beginnings

For much of my professional life as a somatic movement educator and psychotherapist I have been fascinated by the beginnings of life – embryological beginnings, birth and the early development of the infant and young child. I have worked with these beginnings in various ways and contexts, and in earlier chapters some of this was explored. Now, as I approach the completion of my seventh decade of life in this body, thoughts turn more towards endings. My mother, who was my beginning, now calls my attention to the final stages of life.

I have been witnessing her very slow decline as a result of Alzheimer's disease for many years, and most intensely over the last four years. She is now considered to be in the end-of-life stage, though she has lingered in this limbo for some time. It is a devastating illness. Each week it seems I lose another part of the mother I knew as she gradually loses a little more of herself. There is a grieving process that finds no ending as she clings on to life, despite all signs that her brain and body can no longer sustain life. I find a small comfort in the thought that she has had the extraordinary privilege of living her life to its very end. Many people do not have this possibility and are taken too soon, or so it often feels. I witness in my mother, and in other residents of the home where she now lives, a gradual unravelling of the capacities that were developed in infancy and childhood. They travel back through early childhood, into infancy, and come eventually to a place that reflects life in the womb – curled up foetus-like and totally dependent. A life lived full circle – one of the mysteries of life where the body follows the Spirit's return to Source through a reverse journey of the unfolding that happened at the beginning.

Before the pandemic sealed off care homes, virtually imprisoning the residents, I was able to visit for hours at a time and had the chance to witness the ways that the disease affected different people. Drawing on a familiar three-layered map from body psychotherapy, it seemed apparent that once the disease had stripped away the surface layers of social conditioning, underlying strata of difficult, complex and often negative emotions and memories were laid bare. At times it seemed to me that they were re-living early trauma; this is a generation that survived World War 2 as children and, for many, terrifying bombing raids and evacuation from their homes and families, so I can imagine there would be much unresolved trauma in their nervous systems. With the stripping away of social restraints, aggressive and inappropriate behaviour is common, as is anxiety, distress and agitation. I heard lost souls crying out, 'I want to go home' as they wandered up and down the corridors of the care home, not knowing where they were. It seemed to me they were seeking both a return to their childhood home and a return to their spiritual home, to Source or God.

Beyond this stage, for some at least, it seems that a layer of sweetness, an innocence, a light within begins to awaken and be revealed. My mother finally learnt to say those three small words, 'I love you', which had not come easily to her during her long life. She learnt to look me directly in the eyes, which she could never do before. We had moments of intimacy that made the long-drawn-out suffering momentarily worthwhile. On one visit I was touching the side of her cheek, very tenderly, in a way I imagine her mother might once have done, and I saw a tear slide from the corner of her eye. We held each other's gaze and for the first time in our lives I could see her, seeing me. I am here and she is here.

And Endings

My sister's death five years ago was very different. Ill with cancer for several years, she had been able to traverse the path towards her dying with full consciousness, saying her good-byes and finding a place of acceptance. I had the great privilege of being able to stay with her for the last week of her life, sitting vigil by her bedside in the hospice, sleeping alongside her at night as we had done all through our childhood and teenage years.

As her body weakened and gave up yet more of its ability, day by day, my role changed – from tending to basic physical needs and helping her achieve what was still almost within her reach; to what I experienced as *spiritual midwife*, sitting by her bedside, attending to the subtle signs of another gateway passed through. I was reminded of the servant Ninshubur's task as witness to Inanna's descent[2]. Sometimes I sang mantras, silently offered visualisations of Chenrezig's[3] compassionate light, read a poem, held her hand or massaged her feet. For most of the time, simply being present was what was called for. At times I wept quietly, but mostly I would do this outside of her room. I had heard wise teachers say it is important not to cry too much at the bedside of a dying person, as it can make letting go harder for them; this intuitively felt right.

A day or two into my vigil the thought came to me that all the practices I have learnt throughout my life have prepared me for this moment, this work at the threshold, at the bedside of someone dying. My sister.

From somatic work, specifically Body-Mind Centering, I learnt about the physiological functioning of the body, the subtleties of mind and energy moving through soma, the embodiment of self within cells, fluids and tissues, and so much more. Psychotherapy training and practice has given me endless opportunities to be witness to many small deaths and births, as clients made transitions from states of fear and pain to places of inner freedom and flow. From my Buddhist teachers I glimpsed some of the deep and ancient knowledge about the end of life, and learnt some practices to support the passage. Through study and practice of the Discipline of Authentic Movement I have been given the chance to ever deepen my capacity to be *present* to my own and another's experience, to be witness to the expression of the *invisible* through the tangibility of the body moving.

So many teachers and teachings have prepared me for this work that has always been seen, traditionally, as women's work. Just as women are called to midwife infants through the passage of birthing, so too have they been called to midwife others through the passage of dying. The term 'spiritual midwife' came to me while I was in the hospice, and it became clear that this was what was being called for. Intuitively I felt I knew what was needed. I am not trained to do this work – just prepared through decades of embodied awareness practice.

I have 'midwifed' many students through birth processes as part of the IBMT training programme I developed[4]. Just as conception, embryological development and birth have stages that are universal, so does dying. When it is gradual, rather than a sudden or accidental death, able to unfold in what we might call a 'natural' way, we may witness each of the stages that must be passed through. One by one, organ and tissue systems fail and with each, the body loses yet one more function. I witnessed a gradual but steady decline, each day a new threshold passed over, the thread of connection between body and Spirit a little more tenuous. I witnessed phenomena that I had heard my Buddhist teachers speak about – small details that I had barely absorbed, even less understood: it was clear to me that consciousness was leaving her body through an upward movement – from the feet towards the crown of the head. A sequence of painful and uncomfortable physical symptoms unfolded, from feet and legs to lower body organs, through the diaphragm area, then lungs and heart, throat, hearing, mouth. Towards the end an extreme form of mental distress – fear, confusion, disorientation – that the hospice staff named *terminal agitation*, became prominent.

During her final hours this upward movement occurred in a subtler level of energetic change, like a shadow of the physical changes that had just completed. By this time there was no visible movement except the fragile motion of laboured breathing, all other body functions having essentially closed down. Only the subtle, invisible movement of energy, which my somatic practices have taught me to notice, was faintly perceptible and now gradually ceasing; the cessation happened from her feet upwards. I did not have the capacity to see exactly where Spirit eventually left her body, but my attention was entirely focused on her face by this time. In her book *The Soul Midwives' Handbook* Felicity Warner describes this upward progression as the loosening and expansion of the chakras, from root to crown (2013).

I saw how incredibly difficult the process of dying can be. The fear and confusion of the terminal agitation was as distressing to witness as the physical pain that she endured. The hospice chaplain had spoken with us about this stage. He spoke of how the body can be ready to die and the mind and heart might be too, but Spirit struggles to let go of the physical body. What lies ahead is so completely *unknown* and fear might take over. I saw this in my sister: it was so clear that her body could not go on, her organs were failing one by one, beyond recovery; and she had had a long period of preparation, of speaking with family and friends, coming to terms, accepting and finding readiness in her heart for the end. But in the final days a fierce desire to hold on to life took over. The very last words she spoke were 'I want to carry on', as she clung, with a strength I did not know she still had, to the rail of the bed. This was a truly heart-breaking moment for me. In it I could feel all that she still had to give, to receive, to experience in life. She had been practising as a homeopath when first diagnosed with cancer and for the first year after her treatment began; there was so much work still for her to do. She had a husband and two grown sons who still needed her. And so many friends with whom she was engaged in many creative activities. I could feel the promise of all of this, and the pain of it being taken from her, as it must be taken from each of us eventually.

All of this rose up in the space between us to be witnessed one last time, but never to be embodied or fulfilled. I had no wise words or comfort to offer. Had I had a little more presence of mind in that moment I might have said something about her Spirit, her consciousness carrying on, but words failed me. The intensity of the confrontation with the stark and incontrovertible reality of life ending was right there. Dylan Thomas's words, 'Do not go gentle into that good night' (1951) come to mind. We hope and pray that we will go gently, that we will have the wisdom and grace to move beyond desire and attachment to life, to let go, but there is something that seems to underlie and undermine all our conscious intentions – the instinct to survive, to continue going on being, Spirit embedded in the physical body, in love with the tangible matter of sensory life and the web of relationships we have created.

Following those few difficult days there came a time of calm. Heavily sedated now, at the nurses' insistence, my sister finally became peaceful. Despite her mind closing down, it was clear to me that she was still aware of me and would respond with very subtle energetic shifts to my words, touch or meditations. Some part of her consciousness was still very present, despite the dampening effect of drugs on her nervous system. In the last moments there was a subtle but perceptible transformation in her face from an expression of calm to one that I experienced as serenity. She became transparent. An inner light seemed to radiate so softly, quietly, an inner smile shining through translucent skin. She was going beyond, away from us. She took one last faint breath, then her head fell slightly towards me, to her right, as the final breath escaped in three small and quick exhalations.

The precise moment of death was clear, her body now empty of the breath of life, the life force no longer running through it, consciousness moving on. Yet it takes time for the Spirit to completely leave the body. It does not happen suddenly at the moment of the last breath or heartbeat but is a process that takes hours, and some say days or weeks to fully leave. I sat by her bedside for another three to four hours as it was clear to me that consciousness was still leaving her body. The hospice staff had opened the door and windows – they told me they always do this 'to let the Spirit fly free'. What amazing people they are!

A few weeks later, leading my first Authentic Movement retreat after my sister's death, I saw with renewed clarity the phenomenon of Spirit moving through physical matter – the exquisite dance where Spirit meets matter within the cellular, fluid and energetic forms each mover inhabits became transparent in a new way. This experience was intensified, having so recently witnessed the moment when the connection between Spirit and physical body ceased. I had felt this quality of transparency in the days before I went to the hospice too: whilst leading a training group I became momentarily and acutely aware of my own Spirit moving, with such delicate and transparent intricacy, through my dancing limbs. This is life, consciousness infusing matter, and it is beauty.

In my journal, some days after her passing, I wrote:

> *I feel a huge sadness – everything of beauty in this beautiful world will come to an end. Every summer flower will soon fade. Each of us will die, a whole ecosystem closing down and ceasing to exist. One second she was there. The next she had gone. How can this be? The exquisite beauty of life, of people, of flowers and trees, landscapes, sunsets – all of it. All will have to be given up. Her words – 'I want to carry on' – tear at my heart. Of course. We all want to carry on, being in a world of beauty, being a thing of beauty, a creature of exquisite detail and movement that is fine and nuanced, every motion a dance of the Spirit. How could we not want to carry on. The pain of losing all this is so enormous. I can barely breathe with the enormity of it. I can barely hold it.*

And I know that my sister did carry on, in some non-material form within a field of Light.

The words of many Buddhist teachers ring in my ears and fill my heart: everything is impermanent; attachment is one of the primary roots of suffering. Dying teaches us about these truths in a shockingly direct way. And beyond the dying, Spirit continues the dance even as body is returned to Earth and new life grows from it.

[Just a few weeks after I wrote this final chapter my mother died; after many years of illness, in the end her passing was quick and 'unexpected'. I was not able to be with her but a few nights later I had a dream: I was visiting her in a room that was something between a hospital ward and her room in the care home. She was lying in bed as I entered, but as she saw me she threw back the covers and stood up on the bed, reached her arms out wide to her sides, and with an expression of utter joy and freedom on her face and a lightness in her step, she began to skip down the bed like a young child. I knew that she had been freed of the awful illness that had taken her last years, and even the restrictions of her personality had dissolved away. Her Spirit was free to dance and fly away. Her young soul was released.

About six weeks after this my teacher Janet Adler also passed over the threshold of earthly life, into a realm of Light, I am sure. I felt confident that she was well-prepared for this transition after a lifetime of dedicated practice[5]. I offer deep gratitude to Janet for her life and work.]

The writing of this book has been marked by the deaths of two of my primary teachers: Mary just shortly after I began writing, Janet soon after I had finished. Also my sister and mother. In between, the book explores the miracle of new life unfolding. Death and birth eternally cycling in their dance of perfect balance. In the years that my mother was slowly leaving this life and this book was emerging, three beautiful babies, her great grandchildren, were born.]

Notes

Chapter 1

1. Oxford Reference Dictionary. Oxford University Press. 1986

2. https://www.dictionary.com/browse/embody (Accessed April 28, 2020)

3. See the ISMETA website to discover many of these practices: www.ismeta.org

Chapter 2

1. Personal communication during Authentic Movement retreats.

2. http://chesapeakealexander.com/pages/Marsha%20Paludan.html (Accessed January 4, 2023)

3. https://www.apa.org/monitor/oct05/mirror

4. During a Confer talk in London, April 2011.

5. *Somatic imagination* is a term I use to describe a spontaneous and creative unfolding of movement that arises when integrated bodymind is allowed to play and express freely. Following processes where images may offer guidance, there comes a moment when this is no longer needed; the image is released and soma follows its own imaginative pathways. Somatic dance forms such as Release Work invite such flows of creative embodied movement.

6. *Muscle currenting* is a concept originated by Bonnie Bainbridge Cohen that recognises and facilitates optimal muscle function; it describes flows of activation through muscle fibres and their balanced engagement throughout movement. See Hartley 1995 for more details of this and other BMC approaches to movement re-patterning.

Chapter 3

1. The autonomic nervous system consists of two branches, the sympathetic and parasympathetic branches; they work together to maintain homeostasis in the body, help us to meet external challenges and inner needs, and regulate our cycles of rest and activity. This will be explored further in later chapters.

2. This is a phrase Janet Adler has often used in her teaching. I believe I first heard it during an Authentic Movement retreat in Tuscany, Italy, 1993.

3. https://disciplineofauthenticmovement.com/discipline-of-authentic-movement/a-brief-description-of-the-discipline-of-authentic-movement/

4. See https://www.goodreads.com/quotes/1014281-poem-the-spirit-likes-to-dress-up-the-spirit-likes

Chapter 4

1. A phrase used in Buddhist teachings to suggest a quality of pure awareness, all content of thought and expectation stripped away.

2. Michael Soth has written extensively on the objectified body in therapy: https://scholar.google.co.uk/scholar?q=Michael+Soth+on+the+objectified+body&hl=en&as_sdt=0&as_vis=1&oi=scholart

3. See https://www.lindahartley.co.uk/blog.html November 2020: *The Touch of Attention – Somatic practice in hard times.*

4. 'Soul' is another word that is hard to define, and we can find many diverging attempts to do so. At https://www.britannica.com/topic/soul-religion-and-philosophy we read:

*"**soul**, in religion and philosophy, the immaterial aspect or essence of a human being, that which confers individuality and humanity, often considered to be synonymous with the mind or the self. In theology, the soul is further defined as that part of the individual which partakes of divinity and often is considered to survive the death of the body."*

This feels close to my own perspective of Soul as an immaterial essence of our being that partakes both of the rich, heartful, feelingful nature of the individual self (or culture if we are speaking of the Soul of a collective, a forest or a nation for example), as well as having connection with universal Spirit. Soul speaks to the individual (or a particular collective) and Spirit to the universal. If I were to visualise this immaterial essence, I would place it as a connection between the universal and the personal. I see a correspondence with Franklin Sills' description of 'Being': "A locus, or coalescence, of awareness and meaning, the still center in the midst of self-conditions." (Sills 2009: 7) Around this still centre coalesce the archetypal energies, feelings, imagination, creations, and meanings that make us human. Or make a tree a tree, a mountain this particular mountain, or a culture identifiable from another culture – the Soul of the North, the Soul of Africa, the Soul of the Renaissance, the Soul of the Forest.

The reader might have another perspective on the meaning of Soul but perhaps we share a sense that it speaks to deepened, intimate and heartful connection to oneself as well as to the Sacred.

5. More will be said about the Navel Radiation pattern in Chapter 9.

Chapter 5

1. The sources of anatomical and physiological information about embryology that I have used include: Tsiaris & Werth, Martini, Blechschmidt, Nilsson, Bainbridge Cohen, van der Wal (see References for details).

Chapter 6

1. This meditation is drawn from an exercise by Jaap van der Wal during a seminar at the Skylight Centre, London, September 2008.

Chapter 7

1. Bonnie Bainbridge Cohen recognised a pattern of initiation for movements that begin in the head and travel along the length of the spine, which she named the *mouthing* pattern. The opening and closing of the temporomandibular joint (TMJ) sends an impulse into the joint between the base of the skull and first vertebra of the spine. This impulse travels sequentially down the spinal vertebrae to extend or flex the spinal column.

2. There is currently a resurgence of interest in the potential value of psychedelic substances, such as psylocibin, in treating mental health issues.

Research is showing links between mycelial intelligence and enhanced connectivity in the brain.

3. The Institute for Psychosynthesis, London. 1985-7

4. https://www.apa.org/monitor/feb08/oxytocin

5. To draw a timeline, draw a line across the middle of a large sheet of paper, left to right. You might start with conception at the left end and the present moment, or 'the future', at the right. Mark in any way you wish the significant experiences you remember. You can use words, images, add dates, notes about how you felt, etc. Do not worry about all you cannot remember and have no fantasies about – simply include what is accessible for you right now, and see if more memories or thoughts arise over time.

Chapter 9

1. I have written about this in *Servants of the Sacred Dream*, and include sources for further reading there.

2. Some resources for training in somatic trauma therapy can be found here: https://sensorimotorpsychotherapy.org/about/ ; https://sosinternationale.org/se-training ; https://www.moaiku.dk/moaikuenglish/indexenglish.htm

3. A psychotherapist or psychoanalyst using Authentic Movement within their practice might use their analytic skills to elaborate and interpret meaning.

4. I and others have written about this work more fully elsewhere, so I give only brief descriptions here. See Hartley 1995, Bainbridge Cohen 2018, Stokes 2002.

Chapter 10

1. https://www.moaiku.dk/moaikuenglish/indexenglish.htm

2. Jane Okondo describes an integration of somatic movement and bodywork with trauma therapy.

3. Practitioners of Body-Mind Centering and Integrative Bodywork & Movement Therapy are trained to guide students and clients in these movement practices. See www.bmcassociation.org and www.ibmt.co.uk to find practitioners near you, or offering online support.

Chapter 11

1. For a detailed study of the helix nature of the heart muscle, see for example: https://www.sciencedirect.com/science/article/pii/S0022522302001691 or https://core.ac.uk/download/pdf/82548408.pdf Accessed February 16, 2024

2. Please note that the triune brain theory has been challenged and brain function is clearly far more complex than this theory suggests, though it might still be useful as a simplified description. See https://www.ncbi.nlm.nih.gov/pmc/articles/PMC9010774/#:~:text=The%20triune%20brain%20theory%20is,emotion%2C%20and%20cognition%2C%20respectively Accessed February 16, 2024.

Chapter 12

1. https://en.wikipedia.org/wiki/Pangaea

2. https://www.merriam-webster.com/dictionary/intelligence. Accessed May 10, 2021

3. Energy healing and T'ai Chi Ch'uan are two practices that I have found can develop sensitivity to this energetic 'skin'.

Chapter 13

1. https://www.earthrising.one

2. https://www.globaljoysummit.org/summit-home/

3. https://thomashuebl.com/about/

4. https://plumvillage.org/about/thich-nhat-hanh

Chapter 14

1. See for example: https://my.clevelandclinic.org/health/body/23040-endorphins Accessed April 2023.

2. For descriptions of Inanna's journey to the Underworld, the first known recording of the myth of the Goddess's descent, and the place of her faithful servant Ninshubur, see Wolkstein and Kramer (1983); Perera (1981), Hartley (2001); Hartley (2020).

3. *Chenrezig* is the name given in Tibetan Buddhism to an aspect of enlightened awareness, of Buddha-nature, that has the quality of loving kindness and compassion. The *deity*, an expression of Buddha-nature within each and all of us, is visualised and prayed to in order to cultivate these qualities; it is recommended for Buddhists, who do not have special training to work with the dying, to offer the Chenrezig mantra and visualisation for the dying and deceased.

4. See www.ibmt.co.uk

5. See the beautiful film made by Jens Wazel just over a year before Janet's death: "LIGHT – Five Days with Janet Adler": https://www.jenswazelphotography.com/Series/Stories/Janet-Adler

References

Abram, David (1997, 2017), *The Spell of the Sensuous*. Vintage Books

_____ (2020), 'The Ecology of Perception: An Interview with David Abram', Emergence Magazine: https://emergencemagazine.org/interview/the-ecology-of-perception/

Adler, Janet (1999a), 'Body and Soul' in *Authentic Movement*, edited by Patrizia Pallaro. Jessica Kingsley

_____ (1999b), 'Who is the Witness?' in *Authentic Movement*, edited by Patrizia Pallaro. Jessica Kingsley

_____ (2002), *Offering from the Conscious Body*. Inner Traditions

Adler, Janet, with editors Bonnie Morrissey and Paula Sager (2022), *Intimacy in Emptiness – Collected Writings of Janet Adler*. Inner Traditions

Aposhyan, Susan (2004), *Body-Mind Psychotherapy*. WW Norton

Asheri, Shoshi (2009), 'To touch or not to touch: a relational body psychotherapy perspective' in Linda Hartley, *Contemporary Body Psychotherapy*. Routledge

Bainbridge Cohen, Bonnie (1993, 2008), *Sensing, Feeling and Action*. Contact Editions

_____ (2018), *Basic Neurocellular Patterns*. Burchfield Rose Publishers

Barrett, Sondra (2013), *Secrets of Your Cells*. Sounds True

Blechschmidt, Erich (2004), trans. Brian Freeman, *The Ontogenetic Basis of Human Anatomy*. North Atlantic Books

Boadella, David (1987), *Lifestreams*. Routledge & Kegan Paul

Campbell, Joseph (1988), *The Hero with a Thousand Faces*. Paladin, Grafton Books

Carroll, Roz (2009), 'Self-regulation – an evolving concept at the heart of body psychotherapy' in Linda Hartley, *Contemporary Body Psychotherapy*. Routledge

Castellino, Raymond (1995), *The Polarity Therapy Paradigm Regarding Pre-Conception, Prenatal and Birth Imprinting*.
https://castellinotraining.com/special/2011-03-23-Polarity/PolarityParadigm.pdf

Chogyam Trungpa (1975), *Glimpses of Abhidharma*. Shambhala

Conger, John P (1988), *Jung & Reich: The Body as Shadow*. North Atlantic Books

Cooper, Geoffrey M (2000), *The Cell: A Molecular Approach. 2nd edition*. Sinauer Associates https://www.ncbi.nlm.nih.gov/books/NBK9841/

Cozolino, Louis (2006), *The Neuroscience of Human Relationships*. WW Norton

Damasio, Antonio (1994), *Descartes' Error*. Penguin

Davis, Joan (2007), *Maya Lila: Bringing Authentic Movement into Performance*. Elmdon Books

Davis, Madeleine and David Wallbridge (1981), *Boundary and Space*. Penguin

Elisha, Perrin (2011), *The Conscious Body – A Psychoanalytic Exploration of the Body in Therapy*. American Psychological Association

Estes, Clarissa Pinkola (1992), *Women who Run with the Wolves*. Rider

Ferrucci, Piero (1982), *What We May Be*. Turnstone Press

Fischer, Roland (1971). 'A Cartography of the Ecstatic and Meditative States', *Science*, 174 (4012)

Fraleigh, Sondra (2015), *Moving Consciously*. University of Illinois Press

Fulkerson, Mary O'Donnell (1977), *Language of the Axis – Theatre Papers: The First Series: 12*. Ed. Peter Hulton. Department of Theatre, Dartington College of Arts. Available from: https://openlibrary.org/works/OL10589379W/Language_of_the_axis and Triarchy Press (forthcoming)

Gendlin, Eugene (1978, 1981, 2003), *Focusing*. Rider

Gershon, Michael D (1998), *The Second Brain*. HarperCollins

Grof, Stanislav (1985), *Beyond the Brain*. SUNY Press

_____ (1988), *The Adventure of Self-Discovery*. SUNY Press

Grof, Stanislav & Christina Grof (editors) (1989), *Spiritual Emergency*. Jeremy P Tarcher

Hanna, Thomas (1970), *Bodies in Revolt*. Freeperson Press

Hartley, Linda (1995), *Wisdom of the Body Moving*. North Atlantic Books

_____ (2001), *Servants of the Sacred Dream*. Elmdon Books

_____ (2004), *Somatic Psychology*. Whurr/Wiley

_____ (2009) (ed.), *Contemporary Body Psychotherapy*. Routledge

_____ (2015), 'Choice, surrender and transitions in Authentic Movement', in *Journal of Dance & Somatic Practices*, Volume 7 Number 2

_____ (2018), 'Dance in the 1970s – a crucible for *de-schooling*: releasing into being danced', in *Theatre, Dance and Performance Training*. Volume 9, Issue 3.

_____ (2020), 'Woman, Body, Earth and Spirit: Journeys of descent through myth, embodiment and movement practice' in *Spiritual Herstories – Call of the Soul in Dance Research*, ed. Amanda Williams and Barbara Sellers-Young. Intellect

_____ (2020), 'Humanity in a time of Collective Initiation' in *Journal of Dance, Movement and Spiritualities*. Volume 7 Numbers 1 & 2 https://www.lindahartley.co.uk/article_humanity%20in%20a%20time.html

_____ (2022) (ed.), *The Fluid Nature of Being*. Handspring Publishing

Hayes, Jill (2007), *Performing the Dreams of your Body*. Archive Publishing

Holewinski, Britt (online), 'Underground Networking: The Amazing Connections Beneath Your Feet'. National Forests Foundation website: https://www.nationalforests.org/blog/underground-mycorrhizal-network

Johnson, Don Hanlon (1995), *Bone, Breath and Gesture*. North Atlantic Books

Johnson, Trebbe (2018), *Radical Joy for Hard Times*. North Atlantic Books

Juhan, Deane (1987), *Job's Body*. Station Hill Press

Kabat-Zinn, Jon (1990), *Full Catastrophe Living*. Random House

Kern, Michael (2001), *Wisdom in the Body*. Thorsons

Kimmerer, Robin Wall (2013, 2020), *Braiding Sweetgrass*. Penguin

Lake, Frank (1979), *Studies in Constricted Confusion: Exploration of a Pre- and Perinatal Paradigm*. The Clinical Theology Association (available through http://www.bridgepastoral.org.uk)

Lawrence, D H (1928), *Lady Chatterley's Lover*

LeDoux, Joseph (1998), *The Emotional Brain*. Weidenfeld & Nicolson

Levine, Peter (1997), *Waking the Tiger - Healing Trauma*. North Atlantic Books

_____ (2010), *In an Unspoken Voice: How the Body Releases Trauma and Restores Goodness*. North Atlantic Books

Liang, Master T T (1977), *T'ai Chi Ch'uan for Health and Self-Defense*. Vintage Books

Lipton, Bruce H (2005/2008), *The Biology of Belief*. Hay House

Lovelock, James (1991), *Gaia*. Gaia Books

Macy, Joanna & Chris Johnstone (2012), *Active Hope*. New World Library

Martini, Frederic (2001, 1982), *Fundamentals of Anatomy & Physiology*. Prentice-Hall

Montagu, Ashley (1971, 1986), *Touching – The Human Significance of the Skin*. Harper & Row

Mott, Francis J (1959), *The Nature of the Self*. Allan Wingate

Nicol, David (2020), 'Exploring the Subtle Realms – Why?': https://www.gardenoflight.org/forum/2020-03-02/connecting-subtle-realms-why

Nilsson, Lennart (1990), *A Child is Born*. Bantam Doubleday

Ogden, Pat (2006), *Trauma and the Body: A Sensorimotor Approach to Psychotherapy*. WW Norton

Okondo, Jane (2022), 'Somatic Bodywork and Movement Approaches to Trauma' in *The Fluid Nature of Being*, ed. Linda Hartley. Handspring Publishing

Oliver, Mary (1986), 'Poem (the spirit likes to dress up)', in *Dream Work*. The Atlantic Monthly Press

Oschman, James L (2000) *Energy Medicine – The Scientific Basis*. Churchill Livingstone

Pallaro, Patrizia (editor) (1999), *Authentic Movement: Essays by Mary Starks Whitehouse, Janet Adler and Joan Chodorow*. Jessica Kingsley

_____ (ed.) (2007), *Authentic Movement: Moving the Body, Moving the Self, Being Moved - Volume Two*. Jessica Kingsley

Paterson, Jacqueline Memory (1996), *Tree Wisdom*. Thorsons

Perera, Sylvia Brinton (1981), *Descent to the Goddess*. Inner City Books

Pert, Candace B (1997), *Molecules of Emotion*. Pocket Books

Piontelli, Alessandra (1992), *From Fetus to Child*. Routledge

Porges, Stephen (2011), *The Polyvagal Theory*. WW Norton

Postlethwaite, Martha, *The Clearing*. https://allieweigh.com/2018/01/07/4-part-womens-chorus/

Ray, Reginald A (2014), *Touching Enlightenment*. Sounds True

Reich, Wilhelm (1970), *The Function of the Orgasm*. Meridian

Rossi, Ernest Lawrence (1986), *The Psychobiology of Mind-Body Healing*. WW Norton

Rothschild, Babette (2000), *The Body Remembers*. WW Norton

Rust, Mary-Jayne (2020), *Towards an Ecopsychotherapy*. Confer Books

Sager, Paula (2013), 'Witness Consciousness and the Origins of a New Discipline', in *Journal of Authentic Movement and Somatic Inquiry*. Online publication: www.authenticmovementjournal.com

Schore, Alan (1994), *Affect Regulation and the Origin of the Self*. Routledge

Segal, William (1987), *The Structure of Man*. Green River Press

Sheldrake, Rupert (1982), *The Presence of the Past: Morphic Resonance and the Nature of Formative Causation*. Park Street Press

Siegel, Daniel J (2007), *The Mindful Brain*. WW Norton

Sills, Franklyn (2009), *Being and Becoming*. North Atlantic Book

Smith, Dr Tony (1995), *The Human Body*. Dorling Kindersley

Sogyal Rinpoche (1992), *The Tibetan Book of Living and Dying*. Rider

Starks Whitehouse, Mary (1963), 'Physical Movement and Personality', in *Authentic Movement*, ed. Patrizia Pallaro. Jessica Kingsley

_____ (1979), 'C G Jung and Dance Therapy', in *Authentic Movement*, ed. Patrizia Pallaro. Jessica Kingsley

Stern, Daniel (1985), *The Interpersonal World of the Infant*. Basic Books

Stokes, Beverley (2002), *Amazing Babies*. Move Alive Media

Thich Nhat Hanh (2021), *Zen and the Art of Saving the Planet*. Rider

Thomas, Dylan (1951), 'Do not go gentle into that good night', first published in *Botteghe Oscure*, Rome

Tsiaris, Alexander & Barry Werth (2002), *From Conception to Birth: a Life Unfolds*. Doubleday, Random House

Ursell, L K, & J L Metcalf, L G Parfrey, R Knight (2013) 'Defining the Human Microbiome' https://www.ncbi.nlm.nih.gov/pmc/articles/PMC3426293/

van der Kolk, Bessel (2014), *The Body Keeps the Score: Brain, Mind and Body in the Healing of Trauma*. Penguin

van der Wal, Jaap, https://www.embryo.nl/749

Warner, Felicity (2013), *The Soul Midwives' Handbook*. Hay House

Washburn, Michael (2003), *Embodied Spirituality in a Sacred World*. SUNY Press

Weller, Francis (2015), *The Wild Edge of Sorrow*. North Atlantic Books

Wellings, Nigel and Elizabeth Wilde McCormick (2010), *Nothing to Lose*. Woodyard Publications

Whitmont, Edward C (1982), *Return of the Goddess*. Arkana

Whyte, David (2015), *Consolations*. Many Rivers Press

Wolkstein, Diane & Samuel Noah Kramer (1983), *Inanna – Queen of Heaven and Earth*. Harper & Row

Woodman, Marion (1990), *The Ravaged Bridegroom*. Inner City Books

Acknowledgements

My gratitude to all of my teachers over the years, and in particular to the three whose work, described in this book, has most profoundly informed and inspired the development of my own practice – Mary O'Donnell Fulkerson, Bonnie Bainbridge Cohen and Janet Adler.

To all of the students, clients and colleagues who I have met, practiced with and learnt from over the last fifty years, without whom none of it could have been possible. In particular I would like to mention those who have been participating in small group retreats in recent years and whose committed engagement with the Discipline of Authentic Movement continues to inspire me: including Penny, Charlotte, Amy, Paul, Mari W, Rebecca, Brenda, Susanne, Barbara, Melanie, Melissa, Kate, Celia, Nicole, Mari J, Rachael, Sandra, Rosey, Katsura, Dominique, Alice, Graeme, Elaine, Diane, Sudakini, Karen, Louise; as well as the many who have continued to attend the annual summer retreats, despite the setbacks of the pandemic. Small vignettes of some of their practice appears in these pages, and Katsura Isobe and Rebecca Hastings have kindly contributed excerpts from their movement journals.

Several colleagues have generously given their time to read and offer feedback on the manuscript at various stages. To Roz Carroll, special thanks for a detailed reading and review of the whole book as it reached completion; her comments have been invaluable in fine-tuning the manuscript. My gratitude to Cornelia Schmitz who also read the completed book and offered such supportive feedback and discerning questions. Thank you to Penny Collinson, Fran Lavendel and Liz McCormick for their careful reading and comments on sections of the book at different stages of writing; and to Charlotte Darbyshire and Brue Richardson for their positive and encouraging responses.

My deepest gratitude to a few special friends whose constant presence and support has sustained me throughout the writing of this book. With Brue Richardson, artist and healer, I have shared an ongoing 'conversation', via email, over the many miles that separate us. It began as the pandemic began and has been deeply moving and healing; we have shared the highs and lows of this time, as well as our creative work. Brue has kindly given permission to use two of her paintings in the book: "Spring" was begun around the time the pandemic and our extended conversation started, and was completed just as I was finishing the book; "Roots" was created especially for the book when I told her what I was writing about. So both paintings have an intimate connection with this work; I feel honoured to be able to include them.

My wonderful friend Pauline Sayhi and I met regularly throughout these years, walking through all weathers, sharing our challenges and inspirations, drinking coffee on damp logs in wind, hail and rain as the lockdown rules permitted. Being able to share our journeys as we both bore witness to our mothers' decline in the late stages of Alzheimer's was a particular support and blessing.

Liz McCormick, dear friend and colleague, has been a constant source of kindness and a compassionate presence in my life. Even through very difficult times in her own life, she has always been there for me with a kind and wise word, giving attention and love to the details of my life and my writing.

Deep gratitude to my step-sister Gillian Mortimer, who has been like a true sister to me over these years of shared loss and many personal and family challenges. The embodiment of loving kindness, she has been there at every turn of the road. I am thankful too for the presence of her husband Roger, always curious, engaged, ready with a lively conversation and loving support.

Thank you also to Hannah Birley, Cherry Cooke and Melanie Willsher, whose companionship and care during these years of writing has meant the world to me. The walks and conversations have been enriching and sustaining. And to Dave, Joel, Ben, Luca and Alfie for bringing such joy into my life.

A book cannot see the light of day without a willing publisher. Andrew Carey of Triarchy Press welcomed my work with great enthusiasm and a genuine interest in the subject matter, and I am very grateful for his generous 'hosting' of this book. I feel it has found a good home. Thank you to Andrew and the team at Triarchy for their care, professionalism and guidance.

Resources

Institute for Integrative Bodywork & Movement Therapy, which Linda Hartley founded in 1990, currently offers a three-year Diploma Programme in the UK, Lithuania and Russia. The training is an ISMETA Approved Training Programme. For information visit:
www.ibmt.co.uk
www.ibmt.lt
www.ibmtrussia.ru

International Somatic Movement Education and Therapy Association
The professional organisation for somatic practitioners worldwide:
www.ismeta.org

Body-Mind Centering Association
The professional association for practitioners, teachers and students of Body-Mind Centering, founded by Bonnie Bainbridge Cohen:
www.bmcassociation.org

Discipline of Authentic Movement – Circles of Four
A programme of preparation to teach this discipline, founded by Janet Adler:
www.disciplineofauthenticmovement.com

About Linda Hartley

Linda Hartley's career of five decades has spanned the fields of somatic dance, somatic movement education and therapy, and transpersonal somatic psychotherapy. She has worked as a therapist in private practice, as well as teaching independently and for many organisations in the UK and continental Europe. In 1990 she founded what would become a three-year ISMETA Approved Training Programme in *Integrative Bodywork and Movement Therapy*, based on the three foundations of Body-Mind Centering, Authentic Movement and Somatic Psychology.

Throughout her career Linda has authored and edited several books, articles and chapter contributions, the weaving of movement and writing having always been an essential part of her creative work. She now lives in North Norfolk, UK, close to the sea where she grew up.

www.lindahartley.co.uk

Also by Linda Hartley

Non-Fiction

Wisdom of the Body Moving: An introduction to Body-Mind Centering (1995) North Atlantic Books

Servants of the Sacred Dream: Re-birthing the Deep Feminine (2001) Elmdon Books

Somatic Psychology: Body, Mind and Meaning (2004) Whurr/Wiley

Edited Collections

Contemporary Body Psychotherapy: the Chiron Approach (2009) Routledge

The Fluid Nature of Being: Embodied Practices for Healing and Wholeness (2022) Handspring

Fiction

The Broken Line (2015) Elmdon Books

Angel's Wing (in production) Elmdon Books

About Raima Drąsutytė

Raima Drąsutytė is an artist and Integrative Bodywork & Movement Therapy practitioner. Her creative work includes performances, land-art sculptures and drawings from the practices of body movement and touch. Her deep interest is in exploring how art can be a practice/ritual of better connection with the Living Earth and how it emerges and appears from embodied Presence and the felt sense of Interbeing.

Raima lives and works in Vilnius, Lithuania.

dr.raima@gmail.com

Also available from Triarchy Press

Miranda Tufnell
A Widening Field ~ Miranda Tufnell & Chris Crickmay
Body Space Image ~ Miranda Tufnell & Chris Crickmay
When I Open My Eyes: dance health imagination ~ Miranda Tufnell

Sandra Reeve: Ways of Being a Body
Body and Awareness ~ ed. Sandra Reeve
Nine Ways of Seeing a Body ~ Sandra Reeve
Body and Performance ~ ed. Sandra Reeve

Skinner Releasing Technique
Skinner Releasing Technique: A Movement and Dance Practice ~ Manny Emslie

Alexander Technique
Before the Curtain Opens: Alexander Technique in the Actor's Life ~ Kate Kelly

Amerta Movement
The Roots of Amerta Movement ~ Lise Lavelle
Embodied Lives ~ ed. Katya Bloom, Margit Galanter & Sandra Reeve

Somatics and Ecosomatics
Rock Songs: story about walk about story about walkabout story ~ Nick Sales
Suomenlinna | Gropius: Two Contemplations on Body, Movement and Intermateriality ~ Paula Kramer
Attending to Movement ~ ed. Sarah Whatley, Natalie Garrett Brown & Kirsty Alexander
Nature Connection ~ Margaret Kerr and Jana Lemke

www.triarchypress.net/movement